ON BEING A DOCTOR

To Kelly Walton,

Congratulations on your outstanding achievement in Neurobiology, and every best wish for a life marked by professional accomplishment and personal fulfillment.

Best regards,
Joe Corleau

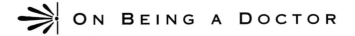

ON BEING A DOCTOR

EDITED BY MICHAEL A. LACOMBE, MD

Published by the American College of Physicians
Philadelphia, Pennsylvania

Designer: Barry Moshinski
Illustrator: Michael McNelly
Production Editor: Amy Cannon Farr

Printed in the United States of America.

Library of Congress Cataloging-in-Publication Data

On being a doctor / edited by Michael A. LaCombe.
   p. cm.
   1. Medicine—Miscellanea. 2. Physicians' writings, American. I. LaCombe,
   Michael A., 1942-   . II. Annals of internal medicine. [DNLM: 1. Physicians—
   Personal narratives. 2. Physicians—Collected works. WZ 112 058 1994]
R118.6.05   1994
610.69'52—dc20
DNLM/DLC
for Library of Congress
Library of Congress Catalog Card No. 94-36460
ISBN 0-943126-65-7

Many of the works included appeared in *Annals of Internal Medicine*, 1990 to 1994.

5 4 3 2 1

TABLE OF CONTENTS

PREFACE

Do art and literature belong in a medical journal? These days, when the acceptance rate for excellent scientific manuscripts hovers at a low 15%, what justification can there be for supplanting research with poetry?

In 1990, Bob and Suzanne Fletcher, then editors of *Annals of Internal Medicine,* initiated the "On Being a Doctor" section to blend with *Annals'* scientific pages more of the spice of humanism than offered by the brief "Ad Libitum" section. No one could have anticipated the response from physician-writers and from *Annals'* readers.

Submissions to the new section came from all over North America, and from Europe, Asia, Australia, New Zealand, and even Africa, with the publication of an especially stirring piece sent from Ethiopia (p. 125). Contributors submitted as many as 15 manuscripts per week—the quality of the poetry has often been astounding, humbling.

Thematic content has covered the entire range of experience of doctoring, from personal illness (an autobiographical account of a physician with HIV infection appears on p. 72) and illness in the physician's family, to the epiphanies and sorrows inherent in caring for others. The most common theme for submitted prose has been the physician's own experience with the dying patient—well over three fourths of all submitted prose, and perhaps half of the submitted poetry. Several remarkable poems deal with human physiology ("The Cell," "The Lungs," "The Nephron"), and a stirring, haunting prose piece covers "The Miracle of the Eye" and gun control (p. 151).

Response from *Annals* readers has been equally impressive. Physicians have been moved, inspired, reaffirmed by these stories, essays, and poems. Patients and physicians' spouses have written, impressed that a scientific journal could find room in its pages for such art and literature. Book agents have called offering to do a collection, something the College has wisely reserved for its own.

The two pieces generating the most mail from *Annals'* readers have been "Who Was Caring for Mary" (p. 35), the harrowing story of an academician's wife suffering from a life-threatening illness, whose frustrated husband finds her surrounded by specialists but without the Oslerian physician they both desperately need, and "Playing God" (p. 83), arguably the most controversial piece, wherein a family doctor covers up a felony-murder for the sake of his patient.

Is there a personal favorite? Yes, there is. "Pathology Report" (p. 63) is a beautiful creation and has a wonderful story to go along with it. When I received the manuscript, I saw it as two excellent poems relating the experience of a miscarriage. The left column is written in strict, anatomical tone, and the right column reveals the woman's own private emotions. Flush with editorial arrogance, I suggested some changes in the last few lines of the right-column poem and sent the manuscript back to the author. She, a nurse in an inner city clinic in Washington, D.C., called me and, meekly, thanked me for the suggestions but couldn't quite see how they would work and asked if I could explain that to her.

"Work?" I asked. "What do you mean, 'work'?"

"Well," she said quietly, "I can see that your changes will improve upon the second poem . . . but then . . . the whole thing no longer reads across . . . ."

I turned quickly back to the poem(s). Immediately, the third poem lifted from the page.

"Oh my God!" I said. "This is incredible."

"Does that mean," came the soft voice, "that you're going to publish it?"

But does literature belong in a scientific journal? There are compelling arguments for both sides of this issue. In this era of mushrooming medical knowledge, how can fiction take editorial pages better reserved for worthy original scientific articles? How can poetry preempt pathology worth talking about? The reasons for continuing with "On Being a Doctor" and "Ad Libitum" go far beyond the mere inclusion of beauty in a journal, as the Fletchers wisely knew. The very act of writing down and submitting such experiences broadens the professional view of the physician. Publication affirms the validity of feelings as having a rightful place still in the practice of medicine—not just for the author, but for thousands of readers as well. And those are data that can never be measured, thank God.

Michael A. LaCombe, MD

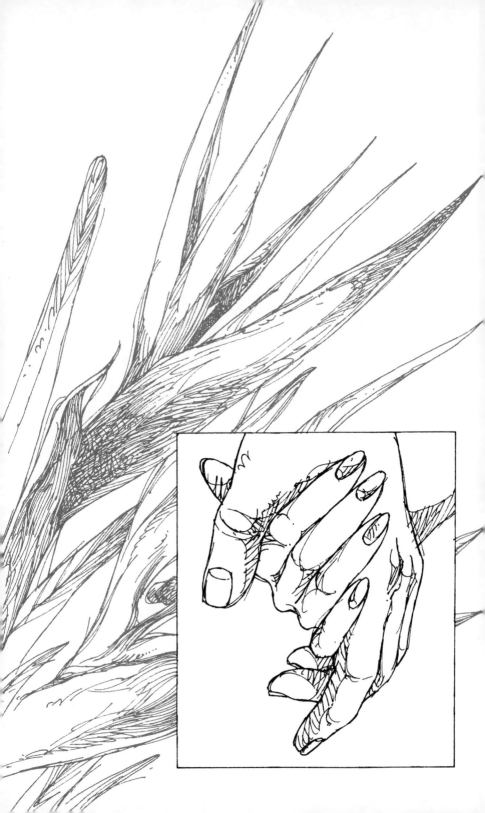

THE DOCTOR TRAINS AND LIVES HIS LIFE

You can soon become so engrossed in study, then professional cares, in getting and spending, you may so lay waste your powers that you find too late with hearts given away that there is no place in your habit-stricken souls for those gentler influences that make life worth living.

Rudolf Virchow

Living the Patient's Story
Michael A. LaCombe, MD

What can we learn from the dying beyond a sudden sense of our own mortality? From the young woman with cancer who, in the midst of her pain and suffering, becomes abruptly still, looks about her hospital room with dawning recognition, fixing her visitors and doctor with a look of wisdom drawn from some mysterious source, and proclaims with certain finality that she loves and will miss them all—is there anything to be gained beyond the poignancy of the moment? Is it that we have become a part of her story?

Or perhaps the patient will be a stern, elderly professor, now close to death. For decades in the classroom, frowning at students over his glasses, guiding them, correcting them, setting them about a proper course, he has secretly wondered whether his life has had any true meaning. And only now, from the steady procession of former students, from the testimony of colleagues and peers, does he gain any sense of consummation. But why only now? Why not 20, 50 years ago, when open-hearted acclamation could have been built upon? Why do we wait until the eleventh hour to speak to our friends from the heart? And even at that eleventh hour, do we ever open ourselves unreservedly? Does it matter?

If it is true, as it most certainly is, that a life in medicine offers the physician a front-row seat in the drama of life, what does the doctor hear in the stage director's urgent whispers, what does he see in the pain of the actor's face, and what can he learn from the troubled eyes of the diva that escapes the notice of those seated less providentially?

A man comes to the hospital to visit his sick wife. Within 2 weeks he himself will die from a mysterious disease. Having cared for the wife, the doctor is asked by her to have a look at him as well. There he stands, a woodsman of enviable strength, unnerved by the pristine antisepsis of the hospital. Behind him, apart and withdrawn, stands their retarded son, in his mid-30s, lurking there by the drapes with feral eyes. He peers at the doctor as though from some dark cave, face expressionless, filling the doctor with an uncommon fear. What begins for the woodsman as fever and troublesome speech, ends 2 weeks later with coma, agonal breath, flaccid palsy, and death. In the intervening days the doctor treats him with rare intensity, calling in the brightest consultants, fine-tuning the delicate machinery of intensive care. The man's wife and daughters hover at the bedside through it all, shocked at the suddenness of his devastation, at this reversal of fortune. She had been the sickly one, and he, her rock, her foundation. Now he finds himself at Death's dreadful door and she will be the one left alone. And through all of the doctor's frantic attention to his father—the urgent summonses to the bedside, the late, sleepless nights before his monitors, the spinal taps and respirator care—the man's retarded son stands silently against the wall and watches. Never altering his stone-like expression, his eyes shift to the nurse running off with an order, now to the doctor's hands probing for hope from his father's body, then to his mother sitting, weeping, and now to his sisters, over-come with emotion, unable to manage their own anger and despair. And in the end, he watches the monitor go straight-line, lifeless, watches a finger flick off the respirator, sees the slow, sorrowful nod to his mother. The man's physician leaves them there with the deceased, and with the nurse, walks out of the room and into the hall, exhausted. There they stand, nurse and doctor, saying noth-ing, each staring off at some point far away. Then the doctor feels something at his arm. He turns to find the retarded man standing still beside him, eyes dark and sad. He has touched the doctor's arm with the point of his index finger.

"Thanks," he says, and walks away.

The nurse, who has seen it all, has seen the wife beatings and child abuse of the metropolitan hospitals, the gunshot wounds snuffing out the life of youth in silly, wanton murder, the nurse who has been hardened by the swirling decay of society manifested by the chaos of the big-city hospital, is overcome.

"Oh Christ!" she says, and buries her face in her hands. The doc-tor fights for control, braces himself against a wave of emotion, and walks her down the hall, holding her tightly.

What has moved them in this way? The wonderful simplicity of the son's gratitude? The startling paradox of a retarded man who seemed to feel the thanks that we often miss? Is there a message here for all of us, buried somewhere in a file marked "What Wasn't Said"? Might it be that we, as doctors, live the case history along with our patients, and too often ignore that role, to our own great loss?

There is in this business of case histories something unique about country doctoring. The rural physician has friends and neighbors for patients, a knife that cuts both ways. On the one hand, the repeated suffering and loss can be overwhelming for the country doctor, and incapacitating for a time. There is the temptation to become jaded, hardened, immune. But the practice of rural medi-cine is enriched by the story of the patient who is your friend, a story the physician lives as well. One often knows the patient first as friend, and his family is an extension of that friendship. The story unfolds. The doctor is part of it.

A young man is electrocuted on a farm. The doctor is summoned to the scene. He is among the first to arrive. He is there just in time to witness the horrible death, to pronounce the patient, and to do little else for him. But the man has a wife. The doctor advises her to remain in the farmhouse, to shun the scene he has had to see, to avoid the nightmares he will endure repeatedly for months. He calls the man's parents, tells them the tragic news. The man's father has a heart condition; that is part of the equation.

The farm belongs to the doctor and the doctor is a friend of the young man's father. They have been fishing companions for 20 years. The doctor, at the request of his friend, had allowed the young couple to rent the unoccupied farm where now his friend's son lies dead. Both doctor and friend suffer terrible pain, an irrational sense that each is to blame for the death of the young man. The farm becomes a forbidden place. The fishing companion stays away. The doctor wonders if he can ever live there, as he and his wife had dreamed. The plot of ground where the electrocution took place remains charred. For two summers, nothing grows there.

And then life goes on. The young wife remarries and moves away. The two friends, doctor and fishing companion, in the serenity of a mountain lake, tell each other of their guilt. They forgive each other, nod to each other down the length of the canoe, and then, flick out their lines to the trout. Later they will return to camp with their catch, gulp cheap red wine from tumblers, and talk about the day. And the doctor will sit back and see himself in life's hard story.

Once, before television and the fast lane, we talked to one another. I like to think that back then, while the rain pounded on the pavement and the elms swayed in protective orchestration overhead, at kitchen tables everywhere conversation swelled with meaning. Phrases like "You really are my best friend" and "Let me tell you how you could be a better friend to me" and "Whatever happens, whatever becomes of you, count on me" were as commonplace as the passenger pigeon. Religion was a feeling back then, not yet relegated to the pitch of Sunday morning TV.

In the country, there are places where these feelings can still be found. And the doctor there is sometimes central to it. He shares with his city colleagues the exciting science that medicine has become. He was trained there. But having camped on a tributary of life's main current, he has avoided much of the consuming business that society has forced medicine to be. Regulation and the paper it breeds, greed and its daughter, litigation, reimbursement and its crafty stalling tactics—all these occupy too much of the city doctor's time.

But there is much that is right with medicine: talking to patients, for example patients who often become friends rather than adversaries and hearing their stories and becoming a part of them. And where the urban academician exerts her skill to empathize with the confused, frightened student, who is heavy with questions and self-doubt, and transforms this fledgling with a few short years of training into a physician of the highest order, the rural physician might teach that student instead to hear from patients what often isn't told these days, and to tell patients what their best friends might have said.

What can we hear in these "case histories"? From a country intellectual, a frequent short-notice dinner companion, and, ultimately, my patient: a learned discourse on nature as Nature, now transformed into life's Path, and then—okay, you win—a fourth, transcendental Dimension which on her deathbed she refers to as He, and corrects with a wink, to She. From a frightened, dying alcoholic who has abused and alienated his family, who themselves now sit in close attention: the rhetorical "is there a god?" transformed into "do you believe in God, doctor?" evolving into "the minister wouldn't bother with me," becoming in the end, a final blessing. From a young girl who has fought Hodgkin disease for 3 years and now lies dying, seemingly defeated: a story about how Heaven will be and how lucky she is to be going there, and how, she says teasingly, with her shy, little-girl smile, I should be going there with her.

Let us allow ourselves to become a part of the case history—a part of the stories in which we may play many roles—stories about that moment of sharing, when all defenses are down, when nothing else matters, when the lines of priority are drawn. That is where the greatest reward in medicine can be found. And the greatest of messages can be found in the patient-doctor relationship at the moment of death. It is a sometimes painful, sometimes joyful message, of missed opportunity and chance occasion, of regret and ecstasy, of guilt and inculpability. It is a portrait of the art of medicine, of that mysterious blend of power and human frailty, and of essential empathy for our fellow man. It is an art all doctors intend to practice, whatever it is that may prevent them in the end from doing so, an art that we, as doctors as well as patients, had better guard against losing.

Flogging Trolls

Chandy C. John, MD

I have sequestered myself in a small room, away from the usual distractions, so that I can sit down and write. I've wanted to write for many months, about many things, but I'm generally most inspired when I'm fatigued and disgusted, so I sleep instead. Not this time—this time I'll write.

I'm doing a combined internal medicine and pediatrics residency and I'm in my 3rd year now, but I took almost a year off last year to do an International Health Fellowship with the American Medical Student Association. I did a half-year of internal medicine as an intern and then to all appearances vanished for a year and a half. Now I've returned, and my fellow diffident interns are suddenly senior residents. The change is remarkable.

I remember my first morning report after I came back from Nigeria; Jeff, who had been an intern with me on the general medicine rotation, was there, and I was glad to see him. He had kept himself dissociated from the medicine game as an intern; he asked questions when he didn't know what to do, he never flaunted what he did know, and he abstained from passing judgment on others. His lack of pretense had made him a pleasure to work with. That day in morning report, he seemed transformed. Now he was the senior resident: citing statistics, firing off questions, quoting journal articles, summarily dismissing others' hypotheses—and doing this more out of arrogance than confidence. It was abundantly clear that the other residents at morning report were impressed by him. They would not have been impressed by the old Jeff, my friend, the quiet intern, but I was, and I found this new Jeff depressing. I found myself thinking, if this is what a good residency does for you, let me drop out now.

It's two in the morning. "What a flog," I say to my intern as I walk into the conference room from a patient's room—and I mean it. This is patient number 10; he has a problem list two pages long with almost every organ system affected, and at this hour of night I'm expected to make him better. I'm going through his history with a fine-toothed comb so I can answer the sometimes inane questions thrown out at morning report. I feel abused. I am sick of answering pages, of writing endless admission notes, of feeling constantly behind, of worrying that I'm missing something important, of ordering unnecessary tests for unlikely diagnoses. But where is the patient in all of this? Is he flogging me? If he is very demanding, he may be part the problem. But more often than not, the patient, his confidence in me, and his strength despite his illness are the things that keep me going.

In our residency the buzzword is "strong," as opposed to "weak." It's macho language, full of sound and fury, signifying nothing.

Anything you disagree with or feel too lazy to deal with is "weak"; anything that saves you time is "strong." We live by these codes, and early on we learn to hide what we don't know, to overstate what we do know, and above all else to be categorical with our answers. There is also a pervasive idea that the only way residents can show how good they are—how "strong"—is to point out mismanagement by the other residents and by the hospitals that have dealt with their patients. People get lost in this maelstrom of rhetoric and pontification; their role in the medical system becomes their definition: a "fascinating" case, a "weak" resident, a "strong" intern.

It's four in the morning. I'm passing by the general medicine team. They're admitting a patient with peritonitis. "It's another dialysis troll,"—the intern says with disgust. That's how they are known— "trolls"—the patients needing long-term peritoneal dialysis who can't seem to stay out of the hospital. The complications of their original disease give them a characteristic appearance: They are small, with short arms and legs, bloated abdomens, and mildly puffy faces, and they are often demanding and rude when they come in. Hence the term "troll"—an unjust, demeaning term. Would we ever say it in front of a patient? Do we really mean it when we say it? I don't think so. It's an expression of our frustration at our lack of a cure, our perception of ingratitude, our exhaustion at four in the morning. And if the patient signs out against medical advice, just when we were getting him or her healthy again, the slur seems justified. How glibly the word rolls off the tongue, not just for noncompliant patients receiving dialysis, but for anyone troublesome. They're "trolls." The 3rd-year students quickly pick up the word. They use it to show that they know our medical terminology. And thus they too become corrupted.

I think of the two interns on my service last month. They were exceptional; they spent hours with their patients and the patients' families, listening to them, caring about them. They knew their limitations, they knew their strengths, and they were honest about both. I found myself praying that they would stay that way, worrying that they would not. It's hard to go through a residency and remain above arrogance and cynicism. The attitudes are pervasive and encouraged. Without brashness and bravado, one's voice is sometimes lost in the chatter. How sad, and how unnecessary. Seeing how patients can suffer because of the complexities of modern medicine, seeing how residents can flourish and thrive in an atmosphere of conceit and pride, we have to ask: Who's being flogged? And who are the trolls?

Concerto

David R. Neiblum, MD

Eyes burning. Always at this time of night. Take the cold, sweating soda can; hold it in turn to each eyelid. Better. Glance out the window. Four-thirty. Darkness.

The ICU lives and breathes around me. A symphony of sounds, smells, movements—machines, and the people to whom they are attached. I drift. My father, taking me (as a boy of 9) to the Young People's Concerts at Lincoln Center. Leonard Bernstein conducting the New York Philharmonic with grace and fury. Crash! screams the cymbal (an ET tube unhooked, the alarm demands the nurse reconnect it). Whisper, whisper from the woodwinds (vents quietly filling a dozen pairs of lungs). Pluck, pluck, pluck of the violin (a chorus of cardiac monitors in various tempos). Guttural vibrations from the bass viola (intra-aortic balloon pump reducing an afterload). *Adagio.*

O.K. Come back now. Keep going. Whose K was low? Right. Murphy. Thirty-three, mother, cerebral bleed, shift, unresponsive on a vent. Husband visiting daily. Talk to him, soothe, explain the procedures, the catheters, the mannitol, and steroids. Change her line, says ID. Maybe she'll wake up (to the nurse). She regards me warily. Keep working—don't think about that. The wire passes easily through the distal port; in slides my new line.

Think I've got someone for you—crashing on 6 South. (The floor resident standing next to me.) Fifties, dialysis patient, febrile, short of breath, hypotensive—probably septic. No access. Grab the triple-lumen kit and go. Trendelenburg, please. A third of the way from the AC joint to the notch, and . . . don't drop the lung. Don't drop it! Hundred percent nonrebreather, and STAT portable chest film on the way. Get him downstairs. Oh, and we'll need a Swan.

Whoosh, whoosh! (an old vent behind me). Drifting again. Wind blowing by the car as we drive to the concerts. He prepares me for the music—explains the meaning behind each piece. The sundry personalities of Holst's "Planets." The thunderous finale of Mahler's First Symphony. Hearing music now—where? Radio blaring by Murphy's bed (husband thought it might help). Listening. Wagner. "Ride of the Valkyries." A fiery, turbulent first movement, but Murphy doesn't stir. Eyes burning, I watch her gently sway with each blast from the vent. *Andante.*

Beeper shrieks. ER. Overdose of Thorazine, alcohol, Valium. Is he tubed yet? Fine. I'll be down. ER's quiet save for the vent alarm. How's your night going, they ask? He's in Trauma/Cardiac 2. Unkempt, poor, schizophrenic, depressed—overdose. I'll save him, though. Ewald, charcoal, vent. Pressors if needed. Mag if he torsades from the Thorazine. Poor guy. Beeper again. Code in the unit. Running up stairs, dizzy, lights rushing, flashing. Faster. Almost there. Almost. Geddings. Seventy-three, end-stage cancer, ARDS, sepsis. Family wants everything done. Everything. Code her, but make it short. V. tach. (*staccato!*). Paddles, please. Clear! Whump! Three hundred Joules rips her body. Flat. Epi, atropine, and over again. Call it, my heart says. Once more. OK, let's call it. Thank you all for your help, but she was . . .

Four weeks in the unit. Three days to go. One more night.

Have to get outside, sit in a garden, an open field. Feel the wind, the reassurance of the sun. Listen to a slow Strauss waltz. Have to see people. Healthy, alive people. People not connected to ET tubes. No A-lines in their wrists. No Swans with their wedge pressures and thermodilution cardiac outputs. No brainstem herniations. No Foley caths, no rectal tubes. No soft restraints.

Twelve more hours before I drive home. An easy dinner, maybe TV, and then sleep. Glorious sleep, free of beepers, and vent alarms. Sleep, free even of dreams, and of music. But not now; not yet. Light glaring in the window—interns will be in soon. Another day of rounds, admissions, transfers, and procedures. Another day hearing the sounds of the unit, which get louder, faster, with the bustle of the morning. Listening, listening. Can you hear them? Slowly at first, then . . . whisper, whisper, pluck, pluck, CRASH!

The third movement's beginning. *Allegro!*

The Cell

Like every reception, there's food
and dancing and bumping
into all those quirky

relatives: blood, Great-aunt Henriette
declares, is thicker
than anything. Family

is in the genes, she says, as if she
just discovered the cell,
the body's time capsule,

recording history for the clumsy, naked
bipeds who hover at
the edge of fire,

evolving into creatures who learn
the cell's workings:
how it sucks up

water from the surrounding matrix
through sticky-lipped
pores; how each tiny

apparatus for food or sex floats
in this one drop of opaque
saline—the primal jelly;

how it composes proteins from
inborn templates for
generations of identical daughters;

how it prepares for the wedding, swollen
chromosomes unwind, line up,
pull to the center and

disperse in their Virginia reel,
mitosis; then the cleaving in two,
the rift, the birth, transformed.

Alice Jones, MD

The Lungs

In the tidal flux, the lobed pair eagerly
  grasp the invisible.

Along oblique fissures, gnarled vascular roots
  anchor the soot-mottled

pulp; pink segmented sponges soak up
  the atmosphere, then

squeezed by the rising dome of the diaphragm's
  brawny bellows, exhale.

Braids of vessels and cartilage descend
  in vanishing smallness

to grape clusters of alveoli, the sheerest
  of membranes, where oxygen

crosses an infinite cellular web: air turns
  to blood, spirit to flesh,

in a molecular transubstantiation, to bring rich
  food to that red engine,

the heart, which like an equitable mother, pumps
  to each organ and appendage

according to need, so even the cells in the darkest
  corners can breathe.

Alice Jones, MD

Predator and Prey
William A. Agger, MD

A rough-legged hawk hangs like a kite on the wind. I watch as he, a more efficient predator than I, hovers effortlessly above broken cornstalks. Rising up and dropping down again, now for a moment he hangs stationary, intent on the ground 20 feet below. Time stops. Abruptly he buckles, for nothing that intense can be still for long. And he is not rising again, so I know that time has stopped for the white-footed deer mouse in his talons. This buteo has come down from the prairies of Canada to feast on my coulee corn-fed mice. It seems to me a long way to travel for this dark predator with his white underfeathers. Dressed in black and white, he wears a perfect suit for a funeral.

And so, I too stalk with hope for a fruitful hunt for ruffed grouse. I'd like to even the score, bird (hawk) kills mammal (mouse), mammal (man) kills bird (grouse). "Fair is fair," whatever that means. However, my footsteps are hardly silent wings, nor can my vision be measured "sharp." Success for this man on this cold January day, too much with snow, too much with wind, seems unlikely. Success for the grouse seems much more likely. It matters not, for I am not in the woods today for success, but rather to be alone.

A dark, sad mood again dropped on me in the office this morning. It came with the fearful face and tearful eyes of a young homosexual. And last month too, it descended with a middle-aged man who had used IV heroin in Chicago. Twelve months ago, it arrived with a young pregnant woman whose lover used the same killing drugs. Twenty-four months ago, it appeared in the apparition of a bisexual business man: "Would the doctor test our baby without telling my wife?"

Not long ago, my subspecialty, infectious disease, was interesting and emotionally uplifting: interesting because of its biology, uplifting because most of my patients could be cured of their infections.

It is no longer that way. Now, a predatory virus stalks humans. It is a cruel, inefficient predator, slowly taking my patients' immunity and then their lives. Given a choice, I would rather fight a pneumococcus, which gives a quick winner-takes-all contest between pathogen and host. A pneumococcus is like a rough-legged hawk; with both, a clean escape can be made.

For a time I escape my morning sadness; a January hunt through the driftless region of western Wisconsin is distracting. Fields, woods, streams, and rivers; all are here to sample. And depending on the sun, or lack of it, and wind, or lack of it, these coulees can be sheltered and warm, forcing my coat open and brimming my hat with sweat. But, out of the ravine and over on the hill to the north, a very cold wind blows.

The human mind is fickle, always wanting new variety, new terrain. That can be in hunt, or food, or drink, or drugs, or sex. This drive for new experience can be our Achilles' heel. It is our cornfield above which our retrovirus hovers. "Should I take the risk? There doesn't seem to be a predator out today," think the mouse and the man.

Today, as I walk, I read frozen tracks of animals in white snow. Fox and rabbit, coyote and turkey, all have gone through their territorial rounds. I wonder where they are now, where they are going. Then, I think of my patients' futures. Where are they now; where are they going? The long-term prognosis is, to use the medical euphemism, "guarded." Seven years untreated? Perhaps, with luck, 14 with treatment? Not much time for these young adults who, until yesterday, had much longer plans.

In 15 years of practice, of treating, of caring, of comforting, there is one thing I have never done. I have never saved a life. I have only delayed deaths. So I help fight this virus with them. It is an emotional fight, a time-consuming fight, and in the end, a painful fight. It is hard to lose young people. My emotions scream, "fair is fair, not this." But I remember the tracks in the snow of the predators and prey. And I doubt grouse think of my predation as "unfair"; instead, they instinctively avoid me.

Suddenly, my thoughts are broken by an explosion of wings as a rusty-feathered blur flushes and flies straight away. It should be an easy shot, and yet, I can't react, surprisingly surprised. It does not seem so long ago that I hunted with quicker strides and more intensity. Then, I would have chided myself for not being alert. Now, smiling to myself, I watched the grouse sail downhill and into the safety of a stand of white pine.

Extremely adapted, the bird escaped easily. But, what of my patients, and my community? We will have to work hard for it. But, unlike other species, we can adapt with our knowledge, warn each other of our common danger, and help each other when illness strikes.

As I look down into the coulee, I find it changing as the midday starkness of black oaks against white snow has softened in the late afternoon light into hues of blue, purple, and pink. It is a familiar place, but I perceive it differently. Pulling two shells from their cold chambers, I drop them into my empty bag and turn toward home and office.

Ceruloplasmin

Among the handful of ocular signs given as jewels
on the day of our initiation—the opacities,
pigments, iritides, cups—we best remember
the only one we will never find, a ring.

It tells this protein's absence. Multiple choice
designed to ferret out what we know about
zinc-collectors or haptoglobin would fail us but
always these blue vowels leap from the

treasure chest of memory. Sky-granted, the name
comes like a password to our tongues whenever livers
scar or limbs leap into fits although none of us,
thinking of it in diagnosis, proves its guilt.

Despite the metaphor our sergeants teach us,
hoofbeats are never horses, and that is why
every patient we see remains a mystery,
a puzzle, exotic, exciting, as nothing is

in the day-to-day, and must have a rare disease
worthy of us who have been anointed and touched
by the serpent's tongue, and given jeweled words
to pass us freely through the temple gates.

H. J. Van Peenen, MD

Monday Morning

In the prelight
A heavy sound from upstairs
I turn from the front door
   to investigate.

My three-year-old son stands
                    naked
   in the soft penumbra of dimmed hallway light
Clutching his favorite blanket
   picture book and well-rubbed panther
            to his chest.
His toes curl on the wooden floor.

I am dressed and beepered—
No snuggling in the warm water bed this morning
   floating back to sleep till sunlight wakens.
Instead, we hug.
I kiss
            his thin neck.
I feel his small breaths.

His bedroom door stands closed,
   heavy in shadows.

At the operating suite,
The residents still at lecture
The patient not yet here,
I enjoy the rote motions—
   follow the green snake tubing to the ceiling
   barbotage dissolving drugs into syringes
   snap open the laryngoscope.

Around me all is bright   pristine   ordered
Primed.
Sterile instruments attend in precise, metallic rows.

I try to recall his just awakened warmth
   in that brief moment
            before

The patient arrives
Naked under hospital issue
Ready to sleep.

                    Audrey Shafer, MD

The Education of a Pathologist
Tsuyoshi Inoshita, MD

*H*ere I was, a pathologist in mid-life crisis. Every goal I had been aiming for seemed to crumble in front of me. I had always been the sort of person who preferred independence and freedom from external restrictions, and thought, as a naive medical student, that pathology would give me such freedom. I would be free of troublesome human relations. But pathology turned out to be suffocating, sterile. I felt constrained. After a few attempts as an attending pathologist in various institutions, I finally returned to clinical medicine. Imagine, a medical resident in my mid-30s! And here I was going back to clinical medicine when so many seemed to be leaving it. I would practice somewhere I dreamed, as a general internist, away from the politics of institutions.

This was arduous, this abrupt transition in my life. My 9-to-5 existence was suddenly transformed into interminable 36-hour shifts. I had no days off. It seemed as though I lived in the hospital. I counted the days until the end of that 1st year. My life gradually improved and I found time to think. I decided to give medical oncology a try. It would be, I thought, the ideal blend of my interest in cancer and my newfound vocation of patient care. I applied for and accepted a fellowship in medical oncology.

Nor was *this* easy. I was a fellow approaching 40 years of age. And on the very first day of my fellowship, I was assigned to the outpatient clinic and saw a small elderly lady in her early 70s. Her name was Mrs. E, and she had just been diagnosed with an extensive small cell carcinoma of the lung. She came with her husband. Their only son, a family practitioner, lived in another large city hundreds of miles away. He never visited his parents anymore. The patient and her husband lived alone, each having the other only for support. Mrs. E was an endearing little lady, and despite her tragic situation, she was stoic and accepting. Her husband was the joke-cracking, jovial type but he couldn't hide his nervousness. I discussed with them the possibility of a good immediate response of her tumor to chemotherapy, but the nevertheless dismal prognosis for long-term survival. Mrs. E agreed to a trial of chemotherapy.

She responded to the medicines quite well. As the treatment progressed I became good friends with both Mrs. E and her husband. They always came together, her husband driving the 45-minute journey from their home, and they were always in the examination room together, smiling, waiting for me. He would tell a few jokes and then leave the room. It was always the same. Mrs. E told me that he was going outside of our smoke-free building to have a cigarette. She didn't confide in me that while she didn't mind dying, she worried about her husband. After six cycles of chemotherapy, she gained complete remission. They were a happy couple again, she cooking for him and he playing golf, cracking his jokes.

Some months later I received a call from an emergency room physician. He told me that Mrs. E was in his department, having been brought in after a seizure, and that her CT scan showed brain metastases. He wanted to transfer the patient to my hospital. When I saw Mrs. E, I was surprised to find how much older she looked, how much more frail. We gave her brain irradiation and started a second chemotherapy protocol. Miraculously she went into a second complete remission. But she knew that this also would be transient, that the inevitable was coming.

"Doctor, I know you can't cure me. Still I worry about my husband. I don't think he can cope without me." I didn't have any words for her, there was nothing I could say.

The encounter became more difficult. Mrs. E and her husband came in with a camera and she took pictures of me. I tried to smile, but knowing the inevitable, fought back the tears. And a few months later, the second recurrence came back as we knew it would and I had to transfer her to a hospice. It was only a few weeks later that I received a call from her husband and was told that Mrs. E had died peacefully at home. I hung up the phone and began immediately writing a letter to Mr. E, telling him of his wife's concerns for his welfare. He responded, grateful for my care of his wife, for my involvement with them and for my communication with him. How bittersweet was this connection and how difficult!

The fellowship is over. The lessons are not. I am a solo oncologist practicing in a small town. There are many Mrs. E's, many spouses similar to hers. Frequently I connect, and too frequently find myself crying inside. But I've not regretted my choice, and feel fulfilled, finally having become a doctor.

On Fainting before the First Pelvic Exam

In the dark,
Her legs in stirrups and draped,
At first furtive glance looking
Like a settee covered for winter,
She was easily mistaken for furniture.

To green-gowned novitiates
The OR was a whirl—
Bottles of blood on the wall,
Sucking, hissing sounds,
And cutlery set at side table—
A ritual in the making.
Heady vapors ablated my smell,
And breathing labored through
The dampening mask.
Glasses steam; two senses gone.

Suddenly that clank,
And with an eerie low hum,
Labial parts flare incandescent,
Strangely disembodied and
Frothy brown with betadyne prep.
Queuing now we wait to press for the
Too large uterus, the possible mass.
Soft belly and searching fingers
Pressing hard enough to hurt,
Except for the anesthesia.

Waiting, the question
Forms itself.
Did she know of our pressing need,
The logic for this occasion?
Was she asked,
And did she also want us?
Players in the spotlight's glare,
Rehearsing now for far-off
Tasks and times,
Tech talk stage left.

Wait.
But why is the air so thin, the
Wait so long in a dizzying dead space?
My turn comes to feel, but
Wait . . . slipping down, hissing all around . . .
Slide back into a gray hollow-headed night.
"Good lord young doctors,"
Says the mother tech,
"One of you has passed!"
Examination under anesthesia.

Thomas S. Inui, ScM, MD

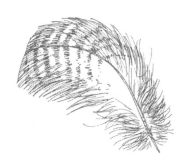

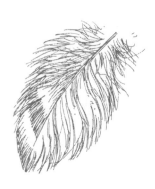

CPR
Clifton R. Cleaveland, MD

The week had been tiring and discouraging—more long-term patients than usual had come to my office with illnesses for which I could do little but empathize and palliate. Aged men and women with fading intellects, emphysemic men slowly fading on continuous oxygen, a young woman with rapidly progressive motor neuron disease—I felt progressively stymied and ineffectual, longing for some more acute situation in which I could work toward a cure.

I sought respite at a weekend showing of the new movie version of *Hamlet*. The reviews had been enthusiastic, and I was prepared for a cinematic treat. Thirty minutes passed, and I was really into the film, marveling at the language, the scenery, and the splendid diction of Close and Gibson. Then a door at the rear of the cinema opened, and an usherette cried out that a doctor was needed. Reflexively, I followed her out. As we rushed to the auditorium next door, I asked what was wrong. She said that a man had been shot. I ran down the center aisle to the side of an old man stretched out supine, apparently having had a cardiac arrest. The house lights had not yet been turned up. *Dances With Wolves* played on the screen. Apparently the old man's collapse into the aisle had coincided with gunfire from the soundtrack. Some of the audience clustered around; others nearby seemed fixed in their seats; most in the full house were unaware of what had happened. An elderly lady wept in an adjacent seat.

He was not breathing. He had no pulse. My reflexes took over as I began chest compressions and directed a nurse who had just arrived to begin mouth-to-nose respirations.

"Call 911."

"We have."

Kevin Costner continued on the wide screen behind us, blurring our boundaries of reality. Another nurse arrived and then a family physician acquaintance. The elderly lady, apparently the victim's wife, sobbed "What will I do, what will I do? We'll have no place to live." I tried to lend comfort as I elicited a fragmentary history from her. He had had a heart attack 5 years earlier, he took digoxin, he had been asymptomatic and active.

"Where's the Rescue Squad?"

"We've called again."

Five compressions and a breath, five compressions and a breath; the house lights slowly came up. His pupils were reactive; the old man began to breathe; he moved his lips.

Our impromptu team was gaining. A firm carotid pulse at a rate of 30 to 40 was present and then faded. I resumed chest compressions while one of the nurses mopped my forehead and helped to remove my sweaty jacket. The family physician spelled me at the chest, and I checked pupillary responses and femoral pulses, now bounding from the closed chest massage. The old man moved his hands—the last spontaneous movement we were to see.

After 20 minutes a fireman arrived with a bottle of oxygen, and I took another turn at the chest—five and one, five and one. The numbing and pounding work of resuscitation continued. Helpful strangers guided the tearful wife away from the circle and tried to console her. From the back door the theater manager announced that everyone should leave and obtain a refund of ticket prices. Many patrons, however, remained frozen in their seats, staring now at the film's buffalo stampede. Perhaps the movie freed them from the horror that all now perceived in the center aisle.

Finally the equipment-laden rescue squad arrived, as did a third physician, who placed an IV in the man's left arm. One EMT inserted an endotracheal tube, while another attached the leads of a cardiac monitor. Coarse ventricular fibrillation. We shocked. No response. Bicarbonate and lidocaine were given, followed by a second shock and another. A junctional rhythm appeared briefly before deteriorating into fibrillation. The electrical and chemical ritual of resuscitation continued against a backdrop of increasing hopelessness. Three doctors, three nurses, and a team of EMTs were powerless to do any more in the theater aisle. We eased the old man onto a board, board onto stretcher, and then stretcher into ambulance. The rescue squad assumed control for the several-mile ride to the nearest hospital. I learned later in the day that the death begun in the theater had ended in the emergency room.

Who was the old man? What would become of the new widow? Who was the retarded adult sitting next to her? A stranger? A kinsman? Why was she worried about losing her home? I knew neither the man nor his wife, yet in the curious way of clinical medicine, a bond of sorts had been struck.

I was weak, sweat-drenched, and utterly wrung out. I wanted to cry. I wanted to know the old man's story. For a brief few minutes our lives had twisted together. I was sharply aware of my own mortality because he lost his life. I felt shaky, decidedly nonprofessional, and vulnerable. I washed up in the cinema's restroom and composed myself. As I rejoined my wife for what remained of *Hamlet*, Mel Gibson delivered the Prince's epiphany to Yorick's skull; words made all the more piercing by the real life just concluded. We viewed the compounded tragedy of the final scene: Gertrude, Claudius, Laertes, Hamlet all dead. Horatio was left to mourn and to struggle to make sense of the calamities engulfing the survivors.

As physicians we see much. Like firemen, things go predictably for us most of the time, and then chaos erupts. At such times we are trained to shift to methodical, automatic countermeasures. Sometimes these prevail. Oftentimes death prevails. Grief erupts and swirls about us. Our job is to try to restore order, to allay somehow the grief and hurt of others. But what becomes of the feelings engendered in us?

The immediate feelings—fatigue, frustration, a sense of aloneness—will fade. Over a longer term we may think that tragedy may broaden our sympathies, but tragedy may also quietly add to our burden of grief, building like charge in an emotional capacitor. Burn-out lurks always, or worse, insensitivity. We try to distance ourselves from the hurt by speaking to colleagues of a failed code or some intervention gone awry. We retreat behind jargon and understatement. Somehow we put the mask of professionalism back in place. We are ready for another day.

The Nephron

You can, with great patience and tiny
tweezers magnified by the dissecting
microscope, lift one away from its home.

There where it lies entangled, with a million
brothers, a million sisters, twisted
together like garter snakes in hibernation,

it busily works with the others, filtering,
reabsorbing, conserving, to such effect
that almost nothing taken from blood

is wasted: sugar, salt, amino acid,
are lost and retrieved like the parable's sheep,
and returned to the joy and welcome of

mammalian flesh. Only what can be spared
is scattered to water and soil
for the nourishment of others, those

small akaryotic brothers and sisters
who branched from the stem before us to dissolve
the Centurion's child, the widow Tabitha.

H. J. Van Peenen, MD

Passing Stones
John W. Burnside, MD

Some doctors practice too long. Some realize it but don't act while others miss the signals, as do their colleagues and friends. I learned that suggesting retirement to a colleague can be as therapeutic as writing a prescription.

Some time ago, I had such a doctor as a patient. He had sent me a few patients for consultation, so I knew who he was from our phone conversations. The patients that he sent did not present particularly difficult diagnostic problems, and I later felt that they had been his advance guard to test the waters. They had in common an intense loyalty to this doctor and spent much of their visits telling me that he was a fine man and had taken care of them for years.

His first visit required several phone conversations between our office secretaries to check, change, and double-check appointment times. Yes, we would be certain to allot enough time. Yes, it would be fine if the doctor told me himself the nature of the visit, and no, we wouldn't do any testing prior to his seeing me. Thank you very much.

That first visit was marked by much bluster and posturing. It seemed he wished to portray that he was very much in control of his own medical condition, was quite knowledgeable, and was seeing me only to confirm the obvious. Later, I was reminded for the hundredth time that things that appear obvious often are not. He had a pain in the neck.

Now this was no ordinary pain in the neck. It had been so troublesome that at times he could not practice. He had consulted famous rheumatologists, neurologists, and finally a neurosurgeon. The first two did not commit, but the neurosurgeon applied his talents. Degenerative joint disease with foraminal encroachment of the cervical roots was the diagnosis. Overgrowth of bone was biting at the nerves and giving him pain—so he was told. He had surgery, was much improved after 6 weeks of convalescence, and he returned to his busy office practice. Now, 6 months later, the pain had returned and didn't I think that a simple injection of steroids into the "trigger point" was indicated?

The examination was not very remarkable. There was some rust on his iron. He was after all well into his 60s, he had worked hard, and a few creaks and squeaks were in order. I could find no evidence of serious disease. "Sure, a little cortisone here where it's most painful won't hurt you and might give you some relief." He seemed pleased that I would take him seriously and that I would concur with his own planned treatment. I guess I affirmed him and he needed that.

He called the next day to share his pleasure that indeed he was better. It wasn't too long, however, until he was back. Many visits ensued, each with more conversation and less therapy. Over the course of time, I learned much more about my medical colleague. He always regarded me as a colleague and not as his doctor. He grew fond of me in a fatherly way and invited my wife and me to visit him at his home.

He was the first doctor in his little rural town, having set up shop just after World War II. As was the case for many doctors of his day, his office and home were one: a large pretty frame house on the main street with the office entrance on the side. There was an astonishing array of lovely antiques, majolica, stoneware, ancient firearms, and bric-a-brac. As he led us on a well-rehearsed tour, he explained that most of the pieces had been payments in kind for services he had rendered to patients. He had been dearly loved. Yet, there was a bitterness in his monologue rather than fond memories of good deeds.

It is a pattern that I have come to recognize. A pattern of chipped enthusiasm, confused needs and wants, and foggy notions of identity. When a new physician starts practice alone, especially as a family practitioner, there appears to be no limit to what he or she can do. Show them that you care, that you are available. Go the extra length and bestow on them the gifts you possess. He had clearly been like this when he started. He recounted wonderful stories of bad-weather house calls, surgery just in time, difficult deliveries, and comfortable deaths, and he told humorous anecdotes about the farm families he attended. He delivered babies at home, took out tonsils in his office, ran office hours well into the evening every night, never took a vacation, and practiced his trade at church and in the barber's chair. There were both smiles and sadness as he told these stories. His sense of personal worth was wrapped in the needs of others. Nothing paid more sweetly than "Doc, you gotta come!" The rule was to never say no. After all, if you don't do it, who will, and someone might die.

So, he never said no. His office was jammed. Appointments that used to be 20 minutes dwindled to 5 or less. Pills from the barrel were dispensed with less care. He had no time to keep up with the literature. "People need me." He would not press for payments so the payments in kind began—first food stuffs and later more substantial gifts.

As time wore on, so did he. The need he unconsciously curried began to wall him in and to become his prison. His jailers, previously friends, never let up. Always calling, always nagging, never understanding that he was tired. "Always thinking of themselves, never considering me" was the last thought before sleep at night. By now the rule DON'T SAY NO was a stone tablet around his neck. Money and material things became the solace for these continual demands. If they were to fillet his flesh, then by God it was going to cost. He accumulated wealth, and bile.

It wasn't evil. It was sad. I slowly realized that what he really wanted from me was a way out. He wanted to quit practice but couldn't bring himself to do it. How do you break the stone tablet that has defined your life for so long? He would be abandoning people, he would be failing, he would be saying "I made a terrible mistake." But, if his doctor told him he had to quit, well what could he do? It wouldn't be his fault and everyone would understand that.

"You know, I think you really should hang it up and quit practice," I said casually one day.

"Quit? I couldn't do that. All those people depending on me," he countered somewhat weakly.

"If you keep this up, you will really get sick and then what use will you be? Besides, there are more doctors around now and your folks will be well cared for. You've done enough. Why not pack it in and enjoy yourself a bit. You've earned it. I'm telling you this as your friend and as your doctor."

"You really think so? I might get really sick? Let me think about that. I just don't know."

That was on a Friday. On Monday, my phone started to ring. When I came back to my office after morning rounds, there were 15 little yellow phone messages taped to my door. Each one from a new patient wanting an appointment. Perplexed, I called the first one.

"Mrs. Stoltzfus, I have your message. What can I do for you?"

"Well, I need some more of those pills that Doc prescribed."

"I don't understand. Why are you calling me?"

"Cause, that's what the note says to do."

"What note?" I asked, getting uneasy.

"Well, there's this note on Doc's door. Says he quit on account of Doctor's orders and if we need anything we should call you at the medical center."

It seemed that he had thought about my suggestion for all of 24 hours. By Saturday he was gone. He and his wife closed shop and went on a 3-month vacation, taking time to put a note on the door of the office.

He passed his stone.

A Cardiac Silhouette Seen on Chest X-Ray

Wampum bag or buffalo head,
A half-deflated basketball,
A fist, a gourd, a sack of seed
Out all night in the rain.

A triangle with corners trimmed,
The sack a Santa carries,
A boy with both knees pulled
Tight up under his chin.

A plum, a pear or mango fruit,
An amber drop, misshapen,
A saddle purse or betel nut,
Walnut in its shell.

A chocolate-covered cherry treat,
The partly open cotton boll,
Gum drop, teardrop, apricot,
Grapes that hang in bunches.

A drawstring purse, fig or face,
The outline of a fishhook,
The summer haystacks by Monet,
Embryo, ellipse.

An uncut gem, an eyeball, egg,
Potbelly stove on legs,
A glob of dough, a dodo bird,
Hard cheese hung at market.

A racket head, a radish root,
A horse's hoof unshod,
A knob, a jug or one wood club,
Water balloon midair.

A garlic clove, a gyroscope,
Marzipan or bassinet
Or listen with your stethoscope:
Bell or bagpipe, castanets.

Phillip J. Cozzi, MD

The Myth of Sisyphus
Joseph Herman, MD

The approach of retirement makes you sentimental. All kinds of things formerly ingrained in the workaholic routine of medicine suddenly take place "for the last time." You begin to welcome and hang on to the few patients who grated on your nerves with perpetual needfulness, seeming ingratitude, and unending attempts to manipulate and load you down with feelings of guilt. They, too, come into the consulting room with a "So you're really going to leave us," making them almost likable, as though they had suddenly awakened to the fact that even a person who got paid for "being there" has some vulnerabilities.

Driving to work, you notice houses, trees, and other fragments of scenery you have passed a thousand times without responding. Late-night reading for pleasure can stir associations never made before. They appear to confirm William James' observation that the greatness of art lies in the vast number of messages people receive from it which the creator did not intend! Most recently, I have been thumbing through *The Myth of Sisyphus* by Albert Camus and, in the author's fire-and-ice world view, I have encountered parallels with my experience as a doctor.

Camus refers to the human predicament as the Absurd, summarized briefly as follows: Because we have the power of reasoning we are forever "outside" the universe, yet there are barriers to rationality that thought cannot negotiate. The only meaningful thing in life is experience, from which a solipsistic ethic and epistemology can be derived. Absurd reasoning demands strained attention to the concrete; it describes while adamantly refusing to explain, rejecting common denominators and according each atom of the universe a "privileged" status. But this approach is precisely the basis of hermeneutics, the phenomenological branch of clinical inquiry that complements what can be learned by the five senses.

One of my greatest regrets is having happened on it late in my career after many patients' "offers" had been ruled out rather than explored. If, as Camus maintains, experience is all, the logic of discarding it just when it can be most useful to others is not altogether clear to me. This does not speak against retirement but points up something of what it can entail. The alternative of continuing to work beyond your time is not a particularly attractive one: haunting the corridors and offices of people whose causes you once furthered, receiving sidelong glances of sufferance and, on occasion, being left behind to inhale vapor trails of passing flattery. I have seen it happen and may have bestowed such a glance myself on an older colleague for which I now ask forgiveness.

Sisyphus is a model for Absurd existence, condemned as he is to move a huge rock up the side of a mountain, only to have it roll back down every time he attains the summit:

> Each atom of that stone, each mineral flake of that night-filled mountain, in itself forms a world. The struggle itself towards the heights is enough to fill a man's heart. One must imagine Sisyphus happy.

I wonder how I will fare in Camus' stony cosmos after divesting myself of both title and authority. Could the two, along with the frenetic daily activity they bring in their wake, have protected me all these years from a flintier reality? I know very well, as Macleish says, how "I have come upon this place." But, at the present juncture, the coda interests me more: "And by what way shall I go back?"

I have often been struck by how fragile are the outcomes we win for our patients. Whether dealing with an enmeshed family or the iron-clad logic of vitamin B_{12} replacement, we can be certain new problems will crop up. Nevertheless, we go through the motions of healing every day, in a sense, raising rocks. Once retired, I shall have no difficulty imagining Sisyphus happy!

Butterfly

Metamorphosis,
I understand
is quite dramatic a change,
yet universal
among butterflies.

Caterpillar, do
you realize
the change as it progresses,
onerous task,
or do you simply wake up
one morning
a butterfly?

Martha Harwit, MD

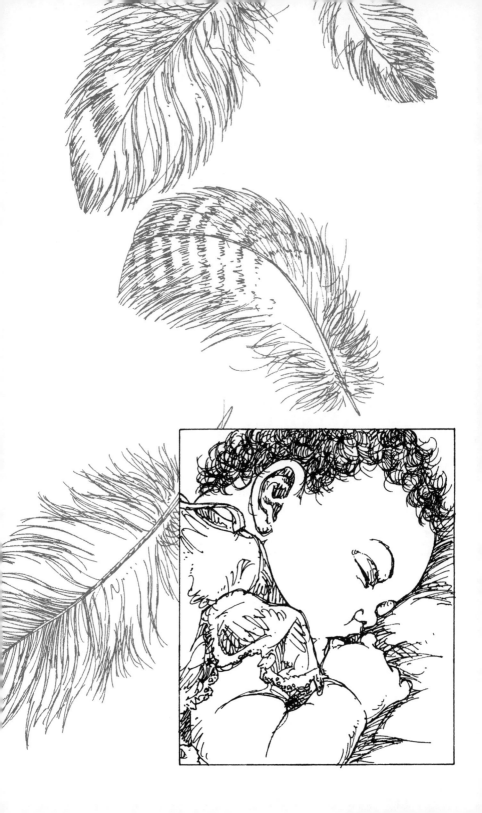

SHE RELATES TO FAMILY AND FRIENDS

If All Who Have Begged Help

If all who have begged help
From me in this world,
All the holy innocents,
Broken wives, and cripples,
The imprisoned, the suicidal
If they had sent me one kopeck
I should have become 'richer
Than all Egypt' . . .
But they did not send me kopecks,
Instead they shared with me their strength,
And so nothing in the world
Is stronger than I,
And I can bear anything, even this.

Anna Akhmatova

Who Was Caring for Mary?

Frederick S. Southwick, MD

*I*t is hard to believe that not long ago my wife Mary was lying in the intensive care unit with less than a 10% chance of survival. How could this be? How could a young, healthy dance instructor and a mother of two children become so desperately ill? The answers to these questions tell us something about how a very healthy, seemingly invulnerable young person can suddenly become extremely ill and can help all of us to understand what can go wrong in our academic medical centers. Criticism of the very institutions that have nurtured me for more than 20 years is difficult. I now see that the lessons learned from Mary's case should be taken to heart by all who wish to return our academic medical centers to their former clinical greatness. I have waited 3 years to describe Mary's encounter with academic medicine. Time and a move to a new university have allowed me to recount my family's experience more objectively. Despite this distance, my story remains a very emotional one. How could it be otherwise? Sometimes a profound personal experience speaks louder than averages, standard deviation, or statistical significance.

The beginning of Mary's symptoms seemed so innocent. She awoke in the middle of the night complaining of burning pains on the bottom of her right foot. Despite aspirin, the pain became sharper and more lightning-like. The next morning, her neurologic exam suggested right popliteal and posterior tibial nerve dysfunction. Could she have stretched these nerves during a straight leg kick at aerobic dance? Why had her symptoms taken so long to begin? She denied having any discomfort during her dances. Pain medications were prescribed.

Mary did not get better. On the 7th day, we saw an academic neurologist who specialized in peripheral neuropathy. Nerve conduction studies revealed marked slowing in the right posterior tibial and popliteal nerves, consistent with a peripheral nerve injury. An MRI of the right leg was within normal limits. I called the neurologist to ask if he had any additional recommendations. Mary's pain was worsening. She was unable to sleep. He stated that no additional measures were indicated and added that he would be away at a research conference for the next week. He suggested I contact him when he returned. Despite several requests that he see Mary, we never heard from or saw him again. His seeming disregard disheartened both of us.

On the 9th day, blue, painless ecchymotic lesions developed under her right fingernail and on the sole of one foot. Later that day her right ankle began to swell. A member of the primary care division ordered a venogram, which demonstrated thrombosis of the right lower venous system and of several small superficial thigh veins. The physician recommended admission but noted that she was not on call and had to pick up her children. I felt abandoned. I had specifically requested this physician because of her excellent clinical reputation, but other concerns clearly took precedence over Mary. I tried to understand. Physicians are too often criticized for not devoting enough time to their families.

Mary was admitted by the on-call attending as a ward case. Admission studies showed an abnormal prothrombin time, an abnormal platelet count, and marked eosinophilia. Was she allergic to the pain medications we had initiated? Could she be allergic to penicillin? (Five days before the onset of her symptoms, she had started penicillin V potassium, which I had prescribed for her strep throat. She had taken penicillin twice before without apparent problems.) Her previous medications were all discontinued and heparin therapy was initiated.

Except for continued leg pain and a temperature of 102 °F, all seemed well until the 5th day of hospitalization. Mary suddenly reported that she felt "a little short of breath" and noted some sharp pleuritic right-sided chest pain. As she was examined, Mary coughed up a small quantity of blood. I thought I was going to faint. A lung scan revealed large filling defects in the right lung and small defects scattered throughout the left lung, a "high-probability scan." Thrombolytic therapy was not felt to be indicated because her heparin doses had been subtherapeutic. This was the first time I learned that her PTTs had only increased to 41 to 42 seconds since admission. Mary was now suffering the consequences of that inadequate therapy as she lay breathless and frightened in her bed.

I rushed to the attending's office. Why had Mary not received appropriate doses of heparin? He seemed unaware of any problems with anticoagulation and pointed out that he had delegated Mary's care to the Senior Resident. He suggested that I speak to the resident. I was welcome to help with Mary's care. Being an academic physician myself, I understood the pressures that her attending was under to maintain his clinical research program while managing patients on the medicine floor. But this was my wife! I became frightened. Who was in charge? More consults were called, but no new therapeutic measures were begun. Her fever persisted and a follow-up leukocyte count was 27 000 with 49% eosinophils.

On the 8th hospital day, Mary developed a new type of chest pain. Her EKG and cardiac enzymes revealed a myocardial infarction! I could not believe it! From simple nerve injury to thrombophlebitis to massive pulmonary embolus—and now, myocardial infarction. Nausea, fear, anger, and sorrow all flooded me with uncontrollable power. I was afraid to leave her bedside. I no longer could remain a passive observer. I reviewed her chart. There had been no mention of the subtherapeutic PTTs in the progress notes before her pulmonary embolus. The laboratory flow sheets had not been filled out. The chart did not contain much of the lab data generated in the last 48 hours. How could the consults or her attending know what was going on? I spent the next 2 hours filling out the flow sheets. Perhaps this act would improve Mary's care.

I again spoke to the attending physician. I pointed out that the rotating intern managing her case was overwhelmed. Clearly Mary's illness was beyond this young man's limited experience. Why hadn't he, as the attending, supervised Mary's care more closely? I tried to contain my anger. A brief look of annoyance flashed across his face, followed by a cool defense of his actions. I quickly realized that further criticism would serve no constructive purpose. Our views of proper medical management were very different. I transferred Mary to the service of a respected cardiologist whom I knew would not delegate her care to the housestaff.

That night they convinced me to leave the hospital. I couldn't sleep. I returned at 2 a.m. and found Mary sitting bolt upright in bed. She had an oxygen rebreather mask covering her face. She was gasping for air! Two hours after I left, she had developed shortness of breath. Her chest x-ray demonstrated near complete opacification of both lung fields. I burst into tears and ran from the room. I couldn't see Mary like this. The grief I felt cannot be explained. I too was hyperventilating. My head was pounding. I whimpered under my breath "Mary, Mary, my dear Mary." If Mary died, what would I do? On my arrival home my father tried to console me. We quickly returned to the hospital. I had to remain strong.

We found Mary sitting up in bed agitated, confused, and markedly tachypneic. Any movement caused her oxygen saturation to drop below 80%. She told me that she was tired and couldn't last much longer. Just before intubation I showed Mary a picture of our two children and told her to keep fighting. We all loved and needed her so much, she just couldn't leave us. She nodded. We looked into each other's eyes as the anesthesiologist gave her an intravenous sedative and intubated her. I realized this might be our last communication. Despite assisted ventilation, Mary's arterial P_{O_2} remained at 45 to 50 mm Hg. She also became hypotensive, requiring vasopressor support with dopamine, levophed, and neosynephrine. Antibiotics and steroids were begun.

As I sat in the CCU waiting room with my brother and Mary's mother, I expected someone to come in at any minute to tell me Mary was dead. I felt like I was sitting in the execution room and that at any minute the hangman would arrive. As I waited, I began thinking of all the wonderful things Mary had done for me and how happy we had been. I thanked Mary's mother for raising such a wonderful person. I realized I should be thankful for the 10 precious years we had had together. Why did God want to take Mary from us? I had no answer. I realized I had to begin to plan for my children's welfare. Would I be able to continue my very demanding academic career? How would I explain Mary's death to my children? The nurse came to the waiting room. I gritted my teeth. She reported that there had been no change in Mary's clinical status.

A critical care specialist arrived that evening. He had just returned from an academic conference. Rather than first going home to see his family, he came directly from the airport to the hospital to assist in Mary's care. The cardiologist, the intensive care specialist, the infectious disease consultant, and the renal consultant all remained at her bedside throughout the night. They discussed together possible management alternatives and carefully planned her treatment. I could see there would be no delegation of care to housestaff that night.

She had failed to respond to diuretics; urine output was less than 5 mL per hour. Arteriovenous hemofiltration was undertaken at 2 a.m. in the hopes of removing fluid. As the renal specialist manipulated the catheter, Mary suffered an asystolic arrest. As the alarms sounded, housestaff from every hospital floor rushed to her bedside. I bowed my head in prayer as they pumped on her chest. I thought as hard as I could, "Please Mary, don't leave me. We need you so much. Don't give up." She didn't. Her heart responded to atropine and isoproterenol. An hour after her cardiac arrest, her urine output suddenly increased; she diuresed nearly 11 liters in less than 24 hours, and her pulmonary function rapidly improved. I knew she would survive. Within 5 days, she was extubated. God, with the help of the physicians in the intensive care unit, had performed a miracle. After a year of convalescence, Mary fully recovered. We have returned to a normal life.

Our experience reveals both the best and worst about academic medical centers. The ability of acute-care, full-time academic physicians to reverse what should have been the fatal complications of her illness, the adult respiratory distress syndrome and profound shock, was truly astounding. However, the care given in the earlier stages of Mary's illness can only be characterized as fragmented and at times impersonal. I was a fellow faculty member. I can only speculate on the treatment an outsider might have received under the same circumstances.

At the onset, I had searched my medical center for an Oslerian physician, someone who could make sense of the complex findings associated with Mary's illness. I found no such physician; instead, I encountered distracted specialists whose actions implied that patient care was of secondary importance. Mary's inpatient attending focused on individual complaints but failed to develop any unifying diagnosis. He ignored small but very important details. This experienced physician admitted to delegating Mary's care to the housestaff. The consequences of that decision reinforce the importance of close supervision. Certainly freedom to help manage patients is necessary for the growth and learning of doctors in training. Should the physician of record abdicate his responsibilities to achieve this goal? Is it no longer necessary for the attending of record to review his patient's laboratory findings and to actively participate in the care of the patient?

Those of us who are academic physicians sometimes forget the sacred trust patients and families put in our hands. We often are more concerned about finishing our papers, preparing for scientific meetings, and completing experiments. Patient care too often becomes an unwanted obligation that is seen as an impediment to advancement. When we are caring for patients, our competitors, particularly those with PhDs, are continuing to advance their research. The competition is intense to maintain funding. Deans are continually re-evaluating our ability to generate research funds for the institution. Rarely are we evaluated on our desire or ability to care for patients.

Many of the older academic physicians bemoan the lack of attention the chairpersons of medicine and the medical school deans pay to good patient care. The skilled general internal medicine diagnostician is an endangered species in academia. Outlying community hospitals now house many of our best clinicians. In many instances, these hospitals may provide better care than their home institutions. When asked directly, department of medicine chairpersons and medical school deans all agree that patient care is important. Actions, however, speak louder than words. Mary's first inpatient attending recently received a prestigious academic promotion. The cardiologist who was instrumental in saving Mary's life has left the university hospital to join a private practice at an affiliated hospital. Patient care is not being rewarded because this activity does not generate research money and does not show up as articles on the curriculum vitae.

The physicians who initially cared for Mary have for the most part forgotten her illness. They were not the ones who had to pay for the oversights in her care. If Mary had died, they would have been able to continue normal lives. My life and my children's lives, on the other hand, would have been irrevocably changed. Being an academic physician with a heavy research commitment, I often worry about my own clinical capabilities. Would I overlook important details under the same circumstances? Given today's academic climate, no one would ever know the difference. We in the academic community, particularly the deans and chairpersons who establish the values and set the goals for our institutions, should remember Mary's illness. My personal experiences have shown me that the top priority for all academic medical centers must be uncompromising and outstanding patient care.

Kath

H. J. C. Swan, MD, PhD

Will you not allow that I have as much of the spirit of prophecy in me as the swans? For they, when they perceive that they must die, having sung all their life long, do then sing more lustily than ever, rejoicing in the thought that they are going to the god whose ministers they are.

Plato
Phaedo

*N*ineteen ninety-two has been a strange year for funerals. Not a heart death among them. Six in all. All solid tumor. Two lungs. Two breasts. A colon. And a cervix. Three men, three women—mean age, 55; range, 34 to 70. Two other physicians, a physician's wife, my accountant of 27 years, a much-loved brother-in-law. And Kath. Katherine Swan Ginsburg, 34, MD, MPH. Department of Rheumatology, Brigham and Women's Hospital, Instructor in Medicine, Harvard Medical School, first author of an article (1) in the 15 December 1992 issue of *Annals*; and my youngest daughter.

Kath had been away from home for 16 years—UCSD, Tulane Medical School, and since 1985 in Boston. Internal medicine resident at the Beth Israel Hospital, fellow in rheumatology at Brigham and Women's. Only when she was dying and after her death did I really have any understanding that she was a mature and truly gifted physician, and could then comprehend not only the tragedy of her passing but the broader loss of a superb role model for young physicians. As a father, I was proud of her coming into our profession, but to me she was still my girl. When I would come to Boston she would get ready to do "The Daddy Thing," she told her friends. Exactly what the Daddy Thing was, none of them knew, but it must have been her way to preserve our father-daughter relationship.

There were 300 or more at the funeral at the Presbyterian Church in Newton, Mass.—enough for a politician or a full professor or even a dean. Patients, nurses, staff, coworkers, members of her church and of her cancer support group, and especially her BI housestaff counterparts—that new generation of physicians that has restored my optimism for our profession. And only then did I understand the maturity she had gained, the respect with which she was regarded, and the sheer love that she had inspired. A BI nurse: "She was a scared intern when I first met her in 1985, but she became a mature and confident doctor quicker than most, and far more compassionate." A rheumatology fellow: "If I wanted to discuss anything, I waited for Kath, even when she was sick, because I would get her complete attention. She'd wait a day or so and then we'd work it out together." A dying Massachusetts General patient with AIDS: "What has happened to Dr. Kathy Swan? She gave me so much time

41

at the BI when I first got sick." Her clinical chief: "We knew that her interaction with patients was characterized by compassion and her respect for their dignity. These qualities have established a standard for all of us to emulate." Dr. H. Richard Nesson, President of the Brigham and Women's Hospital, wrote: "Kathy was recognized as a gifted physician with superb clinical skills and extraordinary compassion for her patients. Her ability to maintain an active clinical practice despite her 3-year battle with cancer was remarkable. The fact that she never let it interfere with her ability to provide care spoke volumes about the kind of person she was . . . . I hope that the establishment of the Katherine Swan Ginsburg Visiting Professorship in Rheumatology will serve as a reminder to us all of an extraordinary physician and a lovely woman."

Kath loved the Beth Israel Hospital. For the first month there were the four times weekly consult calls to the west coast. Then she could sail on her own. "Dad, the only services I didn't like were AIDS and Heme-Onc. So many young patients, and we could do nothing for them." A prophetic statement if there ever was one. Her marriage to Geoffrey S. Ginsburg, now a cardiologist at the BI, on 1 October 1988 was the high point of her life. Her next door neighbor: "After work, they would sit together on the deck with a glass of wine, or iced tea, like newlyweds." Home life was mostly jeans and oversized sweaters. But when the occasion called she was front-cover *Vogue*. A goodly proportion of her BI housestaff were women, and several, as did Kath, married or were married to their contemporaries. This unique group—combining a full professional career with an equally important family life—bonded together in a spirit of total commitment to one another. This support, together with her Christian faith, sustained Kath and Geoff through the horror that they endured for 2 years and 5 months of their marriage of less than 4 years. Fifteen hospital admissions, three laparotomies, two radiation series, three chemotherapy sequences, stem cell transplant, mega chemo, short bowel syndrome, a Hickman and a right nephrostomy catheter for her last 6 months, and countless outpatient visits for radiation, chemo, and labs. And a positive liver biopsy as a 34th birthday present on August 3rd. Yet no complaints, except, in her last elective admission, to gently counsel a new intern because of his audible and inconsiderate comments on her condition. And, between times, back to her normal life, her training— taking boards in rheumatology during chemoradiation, authoring that report in *Annals* before and during stem cell collection, doctor to her patients in the real meaning of that title, and remodeling her home, with the last piece of her new furniture delivered 6 hours after her death.

And what for me—the Daddy; 20 April 1990: "Dad, I don't want to disturb you—it'll be just fine. But I have cancer." My world stopped. At 31, it must be class I. There are so many advances. So much more is known. The old mortality tables don't count. Not for

Kath. So went all of my denials. Her first laparotomy in May confirmed our greatest dread—a single para-aortic node. But chemotherapy was not so different from a decade ago. Radiation therapy did not seem to be effective against the aggressive malignancies. Solid tumor cancer deaths seem to be increasing rapidly, despite all claims of success from "the authorities." In July, the crab took off with incredible fury and was totally unstoppable. Shortness of breath, fatigue, loss of appetite, and intolerable back pain. A CT scan positive for pelvic, para-aortic, hepatic, mediastinal, and pulmonary metastases. And the anger. A Pap smear in 1982: "The cells are seen to infiltrate the adjacent surfaces" . . . in a 24-year-old! She had called from New Orleans: "Everything is okay, Dad, the doctor says I have nothing to worry about."

I returned from Spain on September 3rd, as events accelerated. Turquoise eyes sunken in their orbits. Arm—a stick covered by skin. Pronounced lower limb edema. Severe orthopnea on continuous oxygen consumed all of her energy in the work of breathing. Morphine limited her awareness yet the persona was there. "Hi, Dad, how was your trip? You must be tired." A coughing spell, aspiration pneumonitis, the emergency ambulance to BI, admit to the MICU, chest bilateral white-out. Her friends, coworkers, and the nurses joined in our grief at her bedside. And so, on the morning of the 5th day of September 1992 with Geoff, my wife Roma, and son Jeremy, I watched Kath Swan Ginsburg die, complete with radial line, pulmonary artery catheter, blood gases, and so forth. Knowing the outcome, she spoke her last words before intubation: "Tell them that I'm not afraid"—a final expression of concern and comfort for her husband and family before self.

"Dad, how do I learn to swim with sharks?" asked Kath when offered a staff position at the Brigham in the fall of 1991. She answered her own question: "It's a clinical position, and I'm always comfortable with patients, so I'll just do my best and smile." And the sharks mellowed and loved her. The leadership of the BI and of the Brigham—the institutions that had nurtured her maturing into the person she became—did their part in sharing the economic burden of her illness—she was one of their own, she was family. Her admired coworker and my own dear friend, the respected epidemiologist Dr. Charles Hennekens, wrote to Kath on 1 September 1992, to tell her that her paper had been accepted by *Annals*. He continued: "Your perceptions, sensitivities, dignity and grace continue to inspire us. Contrary to outside opinion, we who have had the pleasure and privilege to know you, also know that Jeremy Swan's greatest contribution to this world was not the catheter but the Katherine." Right on, Charlie.

Reference
1. Ginsburg KS, Liang MH, Newcomer L, Goldhaber SZ, Schur PH, Hennekens CH, Stampfer MJ. Anticardiolipin antibodies and the risk for ischemic stroke and venous thrombosis. Ann Intern Med. 1992;117:997-1002.

Gift at Bar Mitzvah
Charles W. Frank, MD

This brings up the subject of THE THIRD LECH LECHA. This one is from Saba to you, Tavi. Go forth on the journey you described in your autobiography, and get your school records in acceptable shape. With good college grades and your high rating in character, you should be entering the Albert Einstein College of Medicine in 1999. If Hashem and the Dean will permit, I will be there to greet you as you start your medical studies.

This evening, after Havdala, I will give you the stethoscope that I have used for many years. Take good care of it. It is a very fine instrument for examining the sounds of the heart. With study and training and practice, you will be able to learn much about the heart from its sounds.

Recent advances in medical technology have produced many powerful devices and techniques for more precise evaluation of cardiac disease and function. Some of these tests can be quite complicated. Magnetic resonance imaging, for example, requires the patient to be put into a huge device, much as a torpedo is inserted into a torpedo tube.

The stethoscope, by contrast, requires the physician to come to the patient's bedside and connects the ears and mind of the doctor to the heart and soul of the patient. I would hope that this instrument never becomes obsolete and that the beneficial bonding of the doctor to the patient will never be lost.

In the half century that I have been studying medicine, there has been a veritable explosion of new scientific information concerning biological processes and their relationship to human diseases and their treatment. I have been very fortunate to have spent all of my professional life in an academic setting where I could communicate closely with the basic scientists who are the engines of this progress.

As fascinating as discoveries are, we must never lose sight of the fact that the purpose of all of this new science is to improve our effectiveness in caring for patients and in prophylactic measures that may keep us all from becoming patients. This requires a cadre of physicians whose lives will be spent in keeping up with the evolving science while remaining closely and personally involved with the problems facing their patients.

I am thrilled that you have decided to become a doctor. I cannot think of a more useful, interesting, and satisfying way to spend one's life. Enjoy your academic journey! I hope you find it as exciting and rewarding as I have.

Mazel Tov.

The Laying on of Hands
Richard B. Weinberg, MD

g had been dreading the call all day. I was in the library when my pager sounded and, as I walked to the wall phone, I had an ominous premonition. It was my brother. "They found abnormal lymph tissue on the chest x-ray," he said. "What does it mean?" Struck with an upwelling of nausea, I sagged against the wall. Healthy, active, he had gone for the x-ray at my urging, after complaining of fevers and strange chest pains for over a month. "Well, it could be lots of different things . . . ," I began, reassuring him; but I knew. Like my grandparents and sister before him, my brother had lymphoma.

There was much to do. I made phone calls, contacted friends, arranged for a referral to a specialist in his city. I flew down to be with him before his diagnostic thoracotomy. It was lymphoma. A particularly aggressive variety. Together we called home to deliver the bleak news, and the next day I picked up my bewildered and frightened parents at the airport and drove them to the hospital. Together we sat as the oncologists explained the treatment options. When I was not at my brother's bedside, I spent my time in the medical library reviewing the literature and on the phone seeking opinions from prominent experts. In the end my brother chose a new, but promising, chemotherapy protocol at a nearby university hospital and, after the first uneventful cycle, I returned home to work. But every week we would talk on the telephone about his progress, the side effects, his law school classes, life. He achieved a remission that lasted for the summer, and happiness returned to his voice. We made plans for a trip. But then the fevers returned, and he began an inexorable decline, sickened even more by repeated cycles of "salvage therapy." His phone calls came more often and more urgent, and it became progressively harder for me to encourage him and give him hope.

That was when the pain began. I first noticed it as an empty, hollow sensation in my chest at the end of the day. I dealt with it by ignoring it. But as the days passed, the pain became more insistent. It was gnawing and pressing, like a balloon expanding inside my chest. Heartburn, I told myself, and stopped off at the GI clinic to grab some H_2 blockers; but they provided no relief. Stress, I told myself; but neither exercise, nor alcohol, nor attempts to relax made any difference. The pain became constant and kept me awake at night. There had to be an explanation.

Was it angina? A cardiology fellow sneaked me into the heart station one evening and after hours of EKGs, treadmills, and echos pronounced my heart remarkably normal. The pain grew more intense. Maybe atypical pleurisy? I got a chest x-ray in the emergency room and brought it to Radiology. "Lung fields are normal . . . no effusions . . . mediastinum's a bit generous, but it's probably a normal variant," the radiologist on call rattled off before he turned back to his board. The mediastinum is generous?! No! It couldn't be lymphoma! That night I palpated the lymph nodes in my neck, axilla, and groin. They did feel a bit prominent. Soon they became tender, and as the days passed I was certain that they were growing larger. Meanwhile the pain became unbearable. I became obsessed with finding a diagnosis. I prepared a blood smear on myself, and peering down the microscope I saw my death: smudge cells! Leukemia! I grew faint. What will I do? I can't die now! How will I tell my parents? As I panicked, my eye latched onto the tube of blood. A gray top. Fluoride. Metabolic poison. Kills white cells. Pseudo-smudge cells!

In the cold sweat of temporary redemption, I finally accepted the limits of self-diagnosis. I needed a doctor. But who? I knew as well as any informed layperson the names of the experts at our university hospital. But credentials could be deceptive. I had seen them at the bedside, listened to them at conferences, read their clinic notes, and weighed their advice on the wards. So who was the best doctor for my problem? The society cardiologist who couldn't read a cardiogram? The hot-shot oncologist whose housestaff nickname was "mad dog"? The famous pulmonologist who was never in town? If I made the wrong choice, I knew that my symptoms would be zealously pursued with painful tests which, if they didn't disclose a diagnosis, would leave me more miserable than ever. Who? Then suddenly it was clear. Of course! Dr. Davidson!

Dr. Davidson was not a rising star in the Department of Medicine. "I admit he's a very good teacher," the Chief of Medicine was often heard to say, "but he just isn't publishing." "Of course he isn't," one wanted to scream back, "He's out there on the wards every day, like you should be!" And Dr. Davidson certainly tried to be "academic." He was always talking excitedly about his review on gonococcal infections in the inner city. "It's just about finished," he'd cheerfully tell us on rounds, "and it's certainly going to raise some eyebrows." But it never seemed to appear in print. The housestaff didn't care; we loved him.

He was an internist, and at the bedside he shined. It was Dr. Davidson who discovered that an elderly lady admitted three times in 1 month with near fatal status asthmaticus, had recently purchased a new parakeet—and was deathly allergic to it. It was Dr. Davidson who saved a man with tearing chest pain from emergency angiography by pointing out that he had ruptured his pectoralis from an over-enthusiastic weight-lifting session. When the Dean came down with a serious viral pneumonia, it was Dr. Davidson who sat outside his door and fended off the well-meaning

Department Chiefs who descended in multitudes to give conflicting orders to the housestaff. "The Dean just needs to be left alone, and he will get better," he insisted. And he did. And mysteriously, whenever it all became overwhelming and you started to think about quitting medicine, it was Dr. Davidson's arm that came down over your shoulder. "Hey. Let's go down to the doctors' dining room for a cup of coffee," he'd say. You went, and he'd listen, and then it didn't seem so bad.

Surely, I thought, if something's wrong, Dr. Davidson will know. I found him on the wards, told him that I hadn't been feeling well, and asked if he would look me over. He suggested that we go to his office. It was disorienting to be sitting on the other side of the examining table, but Dr. Davidson quickly put me at ease, and soon I was pouring out the whole sorry tale of my chest pain and my brother's illness. It took quite a while. During his physical examination he pored over every inch of my body, felt for lymph nodes, and listened intently to my heart. When he finished, he looked at my chest x-ray and then scribbled a note in my chart. I dressed and, with my heart pounding, turned to face him.

"Do we need any tests?"

"No, I'd say you've done a pretty good job of that," he said with a smile.

"Then you know what's wrong?"

"Yes, I think I do."

"Is it lymphoma?" I choked out, fearing the worst.

"No, your lymph nodes feel normal to me and given the way you've been poking at them, it's no wonder they're a bit tender."

"My heart . . ."

"Your heart is fine."

"Ulcer . . . ?"

"No."

"Are you telling me that I'm imagining all of this?"

"No. The pain is real."

"Then what's wrong with me? What's causing the pain?" I demanded.

"You have heartache."

"Heartache?" The word struck me like a slap to the face.

"Yes. Your brother is seriously ill. You are his best friend, and you've served as his personal physician as well. You've helped guide him to the best treatment, comforted him during the tough times, and given him the strength to go on. You've had to be strong for him and for your family. Now things don't look so good, you know the prognosis of his condition, and you fear what is to come. But no one really understands how much it all hurts you. You love your brother very much, and so you feel his pain in your heart."

Tears streamed down my cheeks. I could not speak.

"It's okay to have Heartache," Dr. Davidson continued. "It's the price you pay for loving someone. And not many of us do as good a job of it as you're doing now, you know." The famous arm came gently down across my shoulder. "Now you keep right on being a good brother and a good doctor," he said, offering me a handkerchief. He sat with me, and after some time I composed myself.

"Thank you," was all I could say.

"You're certainly welcome. We'll talk about things again soon, right? Now, how about a cup of coffee in the doctors' dining room?"

My chest pain eased throughout the afternoon and by evening was gone. Like in the tale of Rumpelstiltskin, once Dr. Davidson had called the name of the demon, its power was vanquished. And although afterwards the heartache returned now and then, I no longer feared it. My brother died 3 months later after a valiant struggle, and I gave the eulogy at his funeral. I finished my fellowship and found a faculty position in another city. I later heard that Dr. Davidson—his magnum opus never completed—was denied tenure and had left the university for another job. I also heard that he was still teaching housestaff and was happy.

In The Oath we swear ". . . to consider dear to me as my parents, him who taught me this art . . ."—and to assist our fellow physicians with every kindness should misfortune befall them. And so it should be. For we carry a special burden: We have learned of the pain that disease brings to mankind and know that often we are powerless to stop it. And when the thin veneer we erect to protect ourselves from this knowledge is shattered, demons that lurk in our minds are unleashed to terrify our souls. In such times we cannot heal ourselves. Rather, in such times, as the Good Doctor Davidson knew, we must heal one another.

Discoveries
Lynn M. Cleary, MD

*A*bigail found the moon last night.

It was a quiet discovery, like most of hers have been. I, on the other hand, heard an orchestra. These are secular miracles to me, her realizations. This one was especially magical because it was so unexpected. Yesterday was full-tilt, non-stop. I finally left the hospital after a late admission and went to pick her up at her grandmother's house; it was quarter till ten when I arrived, and she hadn't been able to fall asleep in her portable crib. She was edgy, of course, as if she resented the fact that I'd left her all day but at the same time resented my intrusion at returning; she'd had her grandmother's undivided attention. Once we were outside she was quiet, attentive. The air was clear and cold, the moon was almost full, and it was surprisingly bright out with all the snow. She pointed up and said, "Deesh?" stared for a moment, then looked at me and smiled with the unmistakable delight of making a connection. All those hours of reading *Good Night, Moon* somehow fit together with her ability to select and then point to something and finally to show me what she had found. We both rode that wave for miles on the way home. Her car seat was near the window, so she could look out and contemplate her discovery. She was quite content with it, checking for its presence at intervals and then just resting or humming with the sound of the motor. The last few miles were along the lake, where the moon's reflection was so lovely. We were both quiet then.

Much of the time my emotions are so private that I'm not certain of them, but motherhood has articulated very clear feelings. I am happy to be feeling what millions of mothers feel, what my mother and grandmother and sister have felt. Part of being a new mother is essentially instinctive, connecting me to ancestors and descendants. Another part is having body and emotions merge, as when milk stains my shirt when she cries. It is hard to describe what it is like to be kicked from the inside out, to nurse, to cry instinctively when she is in pain. I quite like this intimacy.

Motherhood has been remarkable in so many ways; I am only beginning to learn of its effects on me as a physician. It is not just being a patient, going through labor and delivery, healing wounds, or putting up with hemorrhoids. Nor is it learning how to nurse together, mix formula, or figure out if the baby has otitis media. Something in my brain is connecting differently now. Like Abigail, I find things right in front of me that may have been there all along. My neurons are redirected by hormones, my sensibilities have different receptors—more of some, less of others, perhaps new ones. It is not a new language or a different culture, and it is more than a simple renewal.

I have begun to sense that dimension of a patient-doctor relationship that relates to giving in a different way. Traditionally, one thinks of a patient receiving a diagnosis, information, treatment, of a doctor giving care, time, advice. I have been uncomfortable receiving gifts from patients; it was different receiving their gifts as a mother. I must feel motherhood is different from my other roles with them, perhaps more comfortable, perhaps more deserving. Maybe it is the nature of the gifts that made it easy. I have sensed the strength of good feeling when they gave me a blanket, or a rattle, or a bib. Giving gifts empowers the giver, and the usual doctor-patient relationship empowers the doctor in that way. As physicians we assume that power, usually with good intentions, but it does shift the fulcrum of the relationship. It feels very right to readjust that balance, to receive booties, or a stuffed bear, or genuine concern and good will. It feels right to respond to their inquiry about my family, to spend the time sharing that gift of affection. Somehow my child has helped me realize and accept a very important dimension to patient-doctor relationships, before she can even talk.

Another of her silent instructions is to appreciate time. She is my little yardstick, measuring off days and months with each new pound, new skill, new tooth. I am better organized and seem to accomplish more in less time. No doubt there are other ways to learn these skills, but motherhood does hasten their acquisition. Cooking and holding the baby at one time, reading while nursing her—these are good exercises and readily transferable to reading abstracts between returning phone calls at work or eating a sandwich while waiting for the file room clerk to find an x-ray. Although doing two things at once is often necessary at work, it feels more natural now and less of an imposition.

I am also learning to let circumstance direct me. Life is so much easier if I let her show me how she can untie her shoes rather than insisting she keep them on, and much more fun when she chooses between the tambourine and castanets than when I try to teach her a tune on the xylophone. It matters less what antibiotic the resident chooses for treating the pneumonia than that he or she decided to admit the patient for care in the first place at two o'clock in the morning. If Mr. Smith chooses to talk to me about his car mileage and snow tires, why should my own poor sense of timing force him to discuss his wife's terminal cancer that day? There is a time for direction and a time for appreciation. My daughter is helping me sense the difference.

Not long after returning from maternity leave, one of my patients entered the terminal stage of a prolonged illness. She and her husband had been patients for several years, and we had all been aware of the inevitable. Nonetheless, each dying process is a little different, each family circumstance unique. Most physicians process death objectively (write the DNR order, be sure the morphine drip is adequate), but most also occasionally find it jarring, sometimes even unacceptable. This woman's terminal illness was uncomfortable for me. Perhaps it was the juxtaposition of my daughter's recent birth with this patient's impending death, my identification with her as a mother and grandmother, with them as loving parents. It may have been her stoicism, the unfairness of all her suffering.

We were able to have the hospice become involved in her terminal care. During the initial interview among family members, hospice staff members, and me, her husband asked specific questions about how she would die. They were good questions, hard ones to answer, but one of the answers from the hospice in-patient coordinator hit home for me. She explained that patients often labor before they die, just as women labor before giving birth. This patient had been laboring. She had sensed the process and was proceeding with an inner direction. "Don't fight," recommends the labor coach in the birthing classes. Somehow, this process of dying became less uncomfortable for me, and, I think, for the family. The patient had just celebrated a 75th birthday the week before entering real labor. She was ready to labor at the other end of her life. It was less a concept of her leaving than a natural transition from one place to another. The notion of hospice staff working as labor coaches seemed ridiculous, but oddly appropriate, sort of like whiskey and laughter at an Irish wake. No doubt the next of my patients to die will be very different, another disease, a different family. But the concept of laboring as part of dying will now be part of my framework to deal with it.

Motherhood shares so much with the practice of medicine; as Osler described the latter, it is "a way of life." It will be part of my awareness now, an inseparable part of my medical experience. No doubt little Abigail will show me the sun, the stars, and the planets some day.

Working Late

Eight miles east of her, I sit.
The sun is setting off the glass
across the courtyard's grassy width.

"Doctors are hard on their spouses,"
my mother spoke of their constant criticisms,
long, late hours and empty houses

and to me, though in generality.
I thumb through Mr. Martin's chart
and swell with pride and pity.

I know the chart from front to end
and think of how this wall-eyed man
became a kind of patient/friend

before his habits took their toll.
The grubby edge of volume two
has made the bulging binder roll

like the rings in the trunk of a tree,
the dark pulp record of his years.
How balmy was the summer breeze

ten years ago? I bet he knows.
The sun is setting off the glass
and draws the earth along its path

of pink and orange reflection.
The daily tug is pulling in
two opposite directions.

It's time to pull a close to it,
go home to find my breath and strength.
Eight miles east of her, I sit.

Phillip J. Cozzi, MD

On Losing One's Parents
Ken Flegel, MD

My parents are both dead. The fact is neither remarkable nor unique. However, they died within 45 days of one another last winter—uncommon enough to bring me and my family up hard against reality. On the northern tip of Vancouver Island I woke in the dark the morning after the second funeral, my body on Eastern Time, my spirit numb. I made my way back to the village cemetery to say my own private farewell. Douglas firs were silhouetted against the first light of dawn. Colorful funeral flowers had frozen into whited everlastings. I wept into the hoar frost on the new sod and wondered what had become of these lives that had created me. I could not have guessed at the many ways that an answer was to come during the next year.

The first hint came from my children. They could feel my depression the first week I returned and, in addition, had their own sorting out to do. Grandma and Grandpa would never visit again. And if grandparents die, what about parents? "What about you?" they asked. My wife and I answered as clearly as we knew how, reassuring them of our evident good health. That said, confronting mortality became too awesome for them. It was time for the weekly ice-skating outing. I should have understood then, but I couldn't—not yet.

My wife knew, having already been through my experience with her own parents, but she was too wise to say. Instead, she turned my wandering attention to the work needed on our hundred-year-old house and on the garden. The renovations went ahead in good time, but her message was too well coded for me to read.

My first step in understanding came on a camping trip to see the whales on the north shore of the St. Lawrence River. It was July, when the St. Lawrence estuary teems with life. I began to ruminate about the many camping holidays and fishing trips my parents took us on as children. We had had a sensational day spotting the great humpbacks and hearing the visceral sound of their blowing as they surfaced. As I prepared supper, I left the campstove to get some water from the stream. A voice that could only be my mother's made a casual, but not quite distinguishable, comment behind me. I turned to see what she was saying from her accustomed surveillance post at the frying pan. The cruel emptiness hit me again. The next evening the weather became changeable. After supper, I walked away from the campfire's light, gave my nose a satisfying blow, hiked up my baggy trousers, and searched the western sky for clues about the next day's weather. In a flash, I realized I had just recapitulated one of my father's daily rituals. It seemed so suited to me.

Later in the summer, I rediscovered my mother's satisfaction in picking wild berries. Under the shade of poplar trees, I kept my eyes and hands busy collecting the evening treat for my family. In this solitude I began to feel a part of the long tradition of foraging and gathering that had characterized my wandering family.

Autumn came. I screwed up the courage to take out a sweater of my Dad's and try it on. I discovered I was putting on something more than a sweater. My father was somehow with me in that sweater. I wore his aura. In some manner, I became my father.

A neglected memory surfaced, revealing my next step in understanding. Seventeen years ago my wife and I worked in what was then Biafra. The people in the neighboring village buried dead relatives under the floors of the family huts. They erected pink statues of their dead parents in the front yard, a reminder of the life that was. We were living in a culture that was conscious of those who have died, of those who live still, and of those yet to be born; all were part of the psychic here-and-now reality. At that time, our aggressively individuated, Western minds found it merely curious.

Now, I am no longer perplexed by this idea. My parents live on in me. I know what they are thinking. Their life force was passed on to their children. I am one of its custodians; slowly, daily, inexorably, I pass it in turn to my children.

He's Still Alive!

Ted Listokin, MD

*J*ust as an exhausting on-call day is ending, with only enough energy to ponder the slumber that lies ahead, I hear the beeper go off. It is an outside line; the doctor from the intensive care unit answers.

"His pressure has been dropping all afternoon," he explains, "and on maximum vasopressors, I don't expect him to live through the night. You might want to come in now."

I am a bit shaken but not surprised, and, having prepared for this news, I race for the door, purging my mind of the day's events in anticipation of what is to come. In the taxi ride uptown I try to imagine what is happening at the hospital and prepare myself for any scenario. Is he dead already or is he still alive? I chide myself for not having predicted more precisely when things would change for the worse and regret not taking the entire day off to be there and provide support.

I arrive, expecting the worst, and run up the stairs to the unit. A small mob of family is huddled around his bed. In extreme circumstances, the two-visitor-at-a-time rule is mercifully overlooked. He's still alive! Fortunately, I am not too late. Glancing up at the monochrome screen, I see the green tracings of the cardiogram, arterial blood pressure, central venous pressure, pulmonary artery pressure, and respirations that testify to the presence of life in the motionless boy. Motionless except for the chest rising at a mechanically precise rate of 20 times per minute.

His heart rate is 160 beats per minute, his systolic pressure is about 55; at least it will not be long now. Looking around at the family, my family, I sense a collective sigh of relief. The doctor is here. The doctor to whom the entire family turns for advice has arrived. Surely he has brought hope to an utterly hopeless situation. Last year it was grandmother's ovarian tumor, the year before it was grandfather's pneumonia. Now the questions that are literally about life and death concern my young first cousin, barely out of kindergarten for "special" children. I never expected to have close relations as some of my first patients, but by now the terrain has become all too familiar and with each passing year and each new relative I learn to negotiate it a bit more smoothly.

As I take a seat and slip into character, the love and warmth of a nephew gives way to a physician's clinical detachment. They want to know everything and I attempt to explain to father, mother, brother, sister, cousin, and uncle the meaning of the gauges and squiggles. They quickly realize which numbers and lines are important, and follow them. We begin to relax, even to smile, but as the second hour gives way to the third and fourth, the family members notice what I realized at the outset. The numbers are going down, the blips that make up the pressure tracings are shrinking. What will happen in the end is clear to everyone, yet mother and father have declined the offer of a do-not-resuscitate order against the hospital physician's advice and my own.

"He's going to die," I explain, breaking the silence.

"We know, but when?" they counter, almost in unison.

"Soon, very soon," I say, trying to sound reassuring.

The conversation turns to happier times in the boy's life, before the leukemia, before the cardiac arrest. They speak of his smile, of his bizarre fascination with pots and pans when he was 2 years old. They recall an episode of his favorite television show.

When he was diagnosed with Down syndrome shortly after birth, the family grieved. With the support of his parents and siblings and a parade of therapists he reached such a high functional state that he recognized his own predicament and would beg his tutors to "make me smart!" As is common with the disease, he had frequent infections and the family almost lost him to pneumonia very early on. I do not know which played a stronger role in his remarkable recovery, his own indomitable spirit or the unremitting love and patience that his family provided.

Listening to them speak, I think it sounds like a slightly premature eulogy. They cannot let go of him, and when they notice his cyanotic legs they turn to me for an explanation, delaying my own reflections on the imminent death of a loved one so that I can answer their questions.

Just after midnight, my aunt grabs me by the arm and asks that I go with her to speak to the doctor. When I ask why, she says she wants to get an update. An update? Who could be more up to date on the boy's condition than the mother who has spent the last 2 days at his bedside staring at the monitor? Reluctantly, I agree to help her find the on-call pediatric critical care fellow, who has to be awakened from a much needed nap.

"This is my nephew, he's a doctor, so explain to him what's going on."

The introduction embarrasses us both, but the sleepy-eyed man in charge of 12 tiny critically ill patients explains in painful detail the patient's progress. As he reels off numbers corresponding to vital signs and functions, my cousin becomes reduced to creatinine and lactate levels and wedge pressures. I absorb all of the information and make an assessment immediately.

"So?" my aunt asks.

"He's dying. It's only a matter of time now," the fellow replies, echoing my earlier pronouncement.

"But he's a fighter, I know he can pull through."

The fellow looks at me and we share a knowing glance. To be certain, the boy is a fighter. He fought off that pneumonia 3 years ago, maybe he can win this one, too. How does this doctor have the audacity to project so hopeless a prognosis? Whose side is he on, anyway? In my unflagging support for my aunt and family I have lost my sense of reality and objectivity. I catch myself wondering whose side I am on and why I am thinking in terms of "sides" at all. Surely there is no fence between doctor and family, is there?

At three in the morning, his blood pressure drops to below 40 and soon remains in the 30s; his heart rate has dropped to below 130. The hours crawl by as the nurses periodically draw blood gases and give bicarbonate, making sure he does not miss a dose of cimetidine or imipenem. His older sister, who raised him, whispers in his ear and kisses his grotesquely swollen face and hands; I find myself taking more frequent breaks for coffee. Thank goodness he has the chicken pox and we have a private room.

At noon his blood pressure tracing runs flatline, his pulse slows. I join the family in preparing to say good-bye. Mother weeps as father sits in stone-like silence. I call the nurse. She calls the doctor.

He listens to the patient's chest and I feel that my presence is redundant. Even as I hold my aunt I realize that I am a physician also, but without my white coat and stethoscope I must watch from the sidelines, a passive role that is disturbingly similar to the doctor's own. He finishes and shakes his head; there is no pulse and no audible heartbeat, nothing more can be done.

"But he's still alive, look at the monitor," mother exclaims, pointing upward to the screen.

I explain electromechanical dissociation, that the cardiogram tracing will also become flatline soon. We finish crying, kissing, and hugging, and expectantly watch the monitor that reflects a persistent electrical impulse at 95 beats per minute. Two more hours pass, the tear ducts dry, and sleep finally claims me.

I wake up on the floor of the pediatric department conference room and creep back to the unit. He's still alive. Only mother is awake now, holding his pale hand and watching the tracing dance at 1 beat per second.

"He doesn't want to leave us," she says hopefully.

"Yes he does, we just won't let him," I offer, trying to explain to myself my family's behavior.

As a doctor I have explained to the family what is happening to their son as clearly as I know how. Experience with families in the intensive care unit has taught me well. But as family, I am plagued with the uncertainty of what my obligation is and whether it has been fulfilled. I suspect that in the guise of professionalism, I have squelched emotional support to near nonexistence. Does becoming the family doctor make it impossible to serve each role equally? Can the personal and professional be interwoven, or does the part call for a multiple personality syndrome that discerns the invisible signs telling the player which hat to wear? Sometimes it appears that even the simple inquiry "How are you, Dad?" can take on a new meaning and invite responses never offered before I went to medical school.

The monitor starts beeping again, arousing me from self-indulgent rumination. His heart rate is now 60 beats per minute and in a short time the rate drops; the complexes widen and shrink before they disappear, leaving a smooth line. I wait a full minute before calling the nurse. She again brings the doctor, who repeats the ritualistic auscultation.

"I'm sorry. He's gone."

Gone. Dead. Finally, he has died and can rest. The doctor fills out the certificate. The ventilator gently purrs until it is turned off. We watch as the color drains from his face. The paper may certify that he is dead but in our hearts he's still alive.

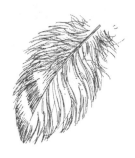

The Good Physician

You and I cannot be friends, for now.
I must coldly probe, pain and score you.
If I care too much,
Yours, and all the others' pains
Will drain, weaken, and kill me.
My love must be shallow enough
For both of us to survive.

Bruce P. Brown, MD

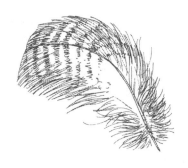

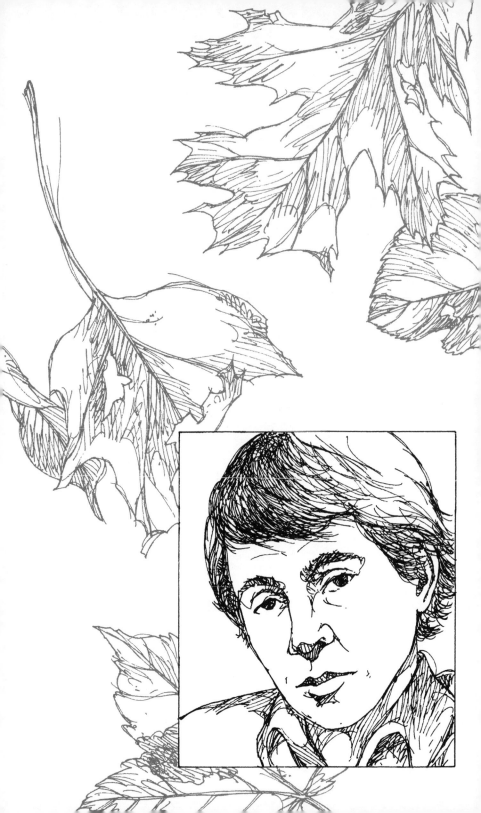

HE DEALS WITH HIS OWN ILLNESS

Les Savants Ne Sont Pas Curieux

Doctors must die, too; all their knowledge of
Digitalis, adrenalin, henbane,
Matters little if death raps again—
Once he may be forestalled, but their great love
Or little love of life is merely human:
Doctors must die like other men and women.

Ah, yes, they know the coronary well,
The lenticulo-striate artery, like a bell
In the village church; and when those strike their knell
What may have been well is no longer well.

Knowledge of nature gives exemption to
No one, his father, and to no one's son;
No one is probably the only one
Who lives any longer than other mortals do.

Merrill Moore

P
A
T
H
R E P O R T
L
O
G
Υ

The specimens	Parts of me
are received	cut from their moorings
in two containers	floating placidly
specimen No. 1	lifted out
labeled	by dispassionate hands
ovary	measured, weighed
the external surface	splayed on a counter
distorted	so much
by a large	once secret
cystic structure	now exposed
filled with	old
dark	imperfections
reddish-brown	festering
material	like a failed heart
specimen No. 2	large, scarred
labeled	utterly useless
uterus	no matter that
opening reveals	a creation of sorts
a mass	suggestive of life
with fleshy-pink	formed
whorled surface	inside
the cavity	which
is compressed	at last
by the mass	cut to the quick
representative sections	proved counterfeit
are submitted	stillborn

Veneta Masson, RN

Heal Thyself

David L. Freeman, MD

 or the physician, the greatest lessons may be found in personal illness. The fear of a steady chest pain, the disability
of musculoskeletal injury, even the discomfort of a short-lived
infection all may bring to the doctor new insights into the
illnesses of his or her patients. But what of major depression?
Can anything more than tragic impairment result from that
experience?

Two days after a routine hysterectomy, my beloved wife
developed fever, abdominal pain, shock, obtundation, and cardiac arrest. Resuscitated, she endured five major abdominal
procedures and, over 6 long weeks, remained barely alive with
ventilator therapy, dialysis, pressor drugs, and cardiac monitors.
She lay comatose, bloated, jaundiced, bleeding. She was
impaled by thoracic tubes, abdominal drains, central venous
lines, arterial catheters, and bladder drainage systems. Would
she live? Would she ever be the same? Would the huge abdominal wound ever close? Would she get AIDS from the blood
transfusions? In time it became clear that my wife would
survive, although the completeness of her recovery would long
remain uncertain. She faced many hurdles of neurologic
impairment, withdrawal from dialysis, weaning from respiratory therapy and tracheostomy, recurrent infection, and wound
closure. After 3 months, she was transferred to a rehabilitation
hospital; 2 months later, she recovered enough function to
allow home care.

In the midst of this disaster, I became aware of a predicament
peculiar to physicians. My wife had had her surgery in the hospital where I am a staff internist, indeed where I had completed part of my training years before. Feeling impelled to rescue
her, I helped to coordinate and to facilitate services, engaged
specialists, humanized her for ICU staff, and kept up on the
details of her therapy. In doing so, I did not permit myself to
show frustration over my wife's tragic outcome; instead, I acted
the role of the concerned, but detached, physician. Moreover, I
maintained the routine at home, comforted my three distraught
children, and continued my office practice for a few hours each
day. However, I was swept with intense loneliness, anxiety, and
sadness, which I throttled. My personal needs were forgotten,
and sleep was impossible.

One morning I realized that I could not read from my
own office notes, that a strange remoteness insulated me
from patients, preventing me from absorbing information.
With the generosity of my partners, I excused myself from the

office for the next 3 months, hoping that I could get a grip on myself.

Now I began to think obsessively, even uncontrollably. I ruminated endlessly on previous periods of minor stress, which now seemed connected to my present emotional state, portraying me as a failure, someone not worthy of living. I became paralyzed, unable to prioritize even the most mundane tasks. I felt no normal emotion, only a diffuse, all-encompassing anxiety that drained me of will and energy. Physical pain afflicted me, and I diagnosed every symptom. When I felt chest pain, I had angina; abdominal pain meant pancreatic cancer; myalgias, fibrositis, and, worst, inability to concentrate became brain tumor. I lost weight, my blood pressure increased, and I felt continuously ill. Evaluations in the emergency room finally convinced me that these were symptoms of depression.

I sought psychiatric help. With psychotherapy assisted by medication, gradually over the ensuing weeks, my sleep pattern improved, my anxiety lessened, and, in small ways, normal feelings began to return. As the depression receded, I realized that I could accurately remember the events, the disordered thinking, and the illness. I began to read about depression and to speak of it with my rabbi. We discussed the nature of family, love, and the human response to suffering in its many guises. I came to appreciate the universality of the experience through which I was passing. I found joy in the mere fact of my wife's survival, and I admired her steadfastness and optimism. I discovered a deeper bond between my family and friends and me. I enjoyed interests long dormant since the beginning of my busy career. I was more aware of my emotional dimensions, my capacity for love, and my life task of nurturing that love.

I returned to the office and to my patients, but with much trepidation. Could I be a doctor again? My patients stayed with me! They were solicitous, kind! I found the time for their own stories, and so much of what they told me was so familiar. Now I listened to tales of emotional anguish. I heard their sadness, their fear, their loss of purpose, their disappointment, and their grief with a newfound understanding. Human distress seemed to find a voice in my examination room where previously it had been muted, expressed only through a filter of common complaints of pain and fatigue. Most important, my responses seemed to find some personal resonance in and even therapeutic value for my patients. And so I learned that illness, even major depression, does not only impair the physician. Indeed, physicians, more than others, are in a position to transform their own pain into healing skills of the highest order. How much we can learn from our own sickness and treatment! I found that I had lived what Rabbi Harold Kushner had written about in his book *When Bad Things Happen to Good People*:

> I am a more sensitive person, a more effective pastor, a more sympathetic counselor, because of [my son's] life and death, than I would ever have been without it. And I would give up all of those gains in a second if I could have my son back . . . but I cannot choose.

The Other Side of Tomorrow
William Paul Skelton III, MD

I was a 33-year-old internist. Life had been good to me. Success, happiness, and love all came to me. It seemed as if it had been too easy, perhaps all too easy. A beautiful, healthy baby boy arrived. Life could not have been better. I had the best of everything.

In mid-1989 my fortunes changed. Slowly, imperceptibly, I began to grow weak. The least physical exertion produced tremendous left shoulder pain. I also developed migraines two to three times each week. Like all young physicians at a medical university, I attributed these symptoms to stress and lack of exercise and sleep. Their persistence, however, forced me to see an orthopedist, who diagnosed left shoulder bursitis. The neurologist diagnosed frequent migraines with aura and started verapamil. The symptoms relented somewhat by late 1989 but soon returned in earnest. My weight dropped 10 pounds. I was perpetually weak and tired.

My wife's birthday was on January 31st and I had intended to take her to dinner. My body had other ideas. I developed hemoptysis, fever, and phlegm. A simple pneumonia, I thought, or perhaps even tuberculosis, either of which needed only antimicrobials to cure me. All I needed was a chest radiograph to confirm my diagnosis. But, as the radiograph emerged from the processor, my pulse quickened and the acrid taste of metal filled my mouth. A large mass filled the anterior mediastinum and left paratracheal area.

I dashed from one benign diagnosis to another. I took the radiograph from the view box and walked outside. My physician-wife was in the hall and asked me how it looked. I could not look at her; I could only mutter that it looked bad. We went into the reading room and placed the image on the viewer. "Squamous cell carcinoma of the lingula," was the calm, indifferent diagnosis offered by the radiologist. But it was me!

All of life's problems pale into insignificance when one is faced with a terminal disease. I felt as if all the burdens of the world weighed on my soul. I couldn't move. I was a participant yet was not really there; it was as if it were an odd dream, a cruel scene in a play I watched from afar. Reality came crashing back when the radiologist asked for some history and my wife whispered that I was the patient. I knew then I was going to die. It was so cruel and so unfair! I had had it all. The list of alternative diagnoses offered by the radiologist could not temper my feelings. I walked away broken, shattered, emotionally destitute.

After facing my own mortality, still I had to tell my parents. I postponed the call, dreading their reaction. I got them both on the line and began to explain the radiograph's abnormality. But I couldn't continue. My heart pounded, my throat constricted, and my eyes filled with tears.

In the days to follow, I ran the entire gamut of emotions. I became convinced that the diagnosis would fit an atypical presentation of tuberculosis. Anger consumed me, and then self-pity. Why me? It was not fair. Self-pity gave way to utter despair. I agonized over my wife and son. Who would teach him to be a man?

I began to bargain with God. "Please make this a treatable disease, and I will do all the right things," I promised.

It came time for the biopsy. As I walked into the CT room, I knew life would never be the same. Whatever the diagnosis, I knew that shortly after chemotherapy would start and I would be less of a person than before. It stunned me as I disrobed and lay on the table. I was a patient!

I was jerked back into reality by the pain of the intravenous needle and I heard a soon to be all-too-familiar line, "Your veins roll." Three additional tries, then success, and the examination began. The tumor was located, the biopsies secured, and then I waited for the results. It seemed that hours passed. The radiologist returned with a presumptive diagnosis of large-cell lymphoma. There I lay, mercilessly perched between the bottomless pit of despair on one side and the faint offer of hope on the other.

I knew it was not the best diagnosis, but I also knew it was not certain death. How do you feel when you are told that you have a slim chance of survival? I was elated!

Within 2 days the hemoptysis worsened. The permanent stains rendered a verdict of poorly differentiated germ-cell carcinoma with seminomatous elements. Chemotherapy commenced immediately. I received a triple regimen of bleomycin, etoposide, and cisplatin.

As I lay in bed on day 1 of cycle 1, I had no idea what to expect. Prehydration and osmotic diuresis produced only the nuisance of polyuria. But when bleomycin was started, all the cruelties of chemotherapy became manifest. I began to shiver, each spell lasting 3 minutes and reappearing in another 10. Then the shivering became worse. My body began to jump and writhe; the episodes were longer, maybe 10 minutes with only 3 minutes off. Waves of heat and cold permeated my body simultaneously. I thought I was stoic, but now I was no longer in control. I was alone in a sea of uncertainty and discomfort.

After the bleomycin came the etoposide and cisplatin and from these came extreme nausea and a visceral retching such as I had never experienced. The inevitable diarrhea only added to the discomfort of total misery. The sight, smell, or thought of food became abhorrent. The mere knowledge that the meal cart was coming produced a return of the retching. I became utterly depressed. I wanted all visitors out of the room. No one was welcome to share my despair—no clergy, no friends, no family. Life held no real meaning. I simply didn't care. My only reality was the clock on the wall. No matter if I slept or daydreamed, there it hung, motionless, watching me.

After an eternity, cycle 1 was over and I could go home. But I could not escape the nausea or the depression. The small pleasures of life were gone. The agony and dread of the next cycle filled their place. At least the migraines were gone.

A radiograph 3 weeks later revealed that the tumor had shrunk in size by more than half. I was overjoyed! Life took on new meaning. I almost looked forward to cycle 2, even with the portocath placed when all my peripheral veins sclerosed.

But my joy was short-lived. The radiograph obtained after cycle 2 revealed no further change in the tumor. My kidneys began to deteriorate and my hearing decreased, further obscured by tinnitus. I began to lose my hair. Each morning I would awaken to a pillow case covered with hair. The shower drain would clog with it. Now, as I looked in the mirror at my balding head, my sunken eyes, and my emaciated body, I knew I might not survive. The thought of that parasite of my own body, sucking the vital essence of my being, revolted me. How could I persist in nourishing this unwelcome intruder? How could I get rid of it?

Cycle 3 came and went. The decision was made to proceed with a thoracotomy because the radiograph revealed no further change in size. They talked of postoperative radiotherapy. Even if I survived, what would be left of me? The bleomycin had ruined my lungs. The cisplatin had irreversibly damaged my kidneys, my hearing, and the sensation in my feet. I decided against cycle 4. If I had such an arduous road to travel, why augment the present damage? My wife insisted and convinced me to proceed.

The day of the thoracotomy arrived. I greeted it with no emotion. I was a prisoner. I had no way to turn. My life was in the hands of the surgeon and God.

Stabbing chest pain awakened me several hours later in the surgical intensive care unit. It would not be discovered until 12 hours later that the epidural catheter for postoperative analgesia was malpositioned, and I had been given no pain relief. During this time of lancinating pain, my `wife appeared at my bedside. Her voice was sweet as honeydew, and her message was one of victory: No viable cancer cells were seen in any of the sections—no more tumor!

With such news, I could easily tolerate the next several days. Nothing seemed to bother me anymore, not the incessant examinations by the 3rd-year medical students, not even the nurse awaking me at two o'clock in the morning to see if I was asleep. All of this became insignificant as I realized I had won.

Looking at my body in the mirror, I could see the ravages of the battle that I had just been through. The midsternal scar was beginning to heal. Another ugly reminder was the portocath under my left clavicle. My oncologist suggested we remove the portocath; it was no longer needed.

The nightmare would not be over quite as quickly as I had hoped. During removal of the portocath, the dissecting blade sheared 7 inches of tubing. This 7 inches migrated into the right ventricle and promptly caused bursts of ventricular ectopy. How could this happen to me? After all I had been through, after all the chemotherapy, the pain and anguish of the thoracotomy, was I to die from a ventricular arrhythmia due to a silly mistake like this? Was I going to be allowed to run the entire marathon, only to collapse within sight of the finish line? Fortunately, an experienced angiographer was able to access the right femoral vein and hook this unwelcome piece of tubing and end my nightmare.

It has now been 3 years since diagnosis. All post-procedural examinations have been within normal limits. I was given the unique opportunity to see life from various extremes. Being a patient was terribly unpleasant. I know how my patients feel. I know that there is much more to being a good physician than just being a good diagnostician. I have learned empathy and compassion. Facing death itself produced an awareness of my own mortality I will never forget.

Doctors at Lunch

I knew something went wrong that day
Jerry told us doctors at lunch
he hadn't enjoyed Costa Rica. After all,
trailblazer is his part in our days—
dialyzing nephrons, skiing Crystal,
priming the Staff for peer review.
Most Wednesdays, he scales a Cascade.

A month later the nurses phone—
they'd found him lost in a patient's room
leafing aimlessly through the chart.
Drugs? Hardly. He thrives on competition.
Depression? A malpractice suit taking its toll?
A Glioblastoma stealing zest, misdirecting?
An MRI reveals the cause. "Too soon," we groan.
Every now and then, one of us will sigh
for our colleague (finished radiation,
a second debulking, going with family to Kauai).
Mostly we complain about the S&L, Medicare;
share stories—patients, Boards, kids, cars;
laugh; critique restaurants, movies,
one or another's choice of tie.

In silence, we calculate time.
We all know it will take ten lifetimes
to answer every beckoning, snow-capped peak,
inhale deeply every purpled alpine meadow,
clear our brains in just one of those cool
pristine lakes Jerry told us about,
after a long hot climb.

John L. Wright, MD

From the Eye of the Storm, with the Eyes of a Physician

Hacib Aoun, MD

*D*r. Rabin, a renowned endocrinologist, was stricken by amyotrophic lateral sclerosis in 1979 at the age of 45 years. Although the illness eventually took his life, it never took away his determination or his dignity. When the illness made it difficult for him to walk, he used a cane and came to work. When the illness made the cane insufficient, he used a wheelchair and kept coming to work. And even when the illness took away from him the ability to speak, he continued to communicate with the assistance of a computer that would select words and letters by the movement of his eyes. He conceded nothing to his illness. He continued to raise an admirable family and, despite all the impositions of the illness, he struggled to maintain for them a normal life. However, after he became a patient, he often faced a side of medicine that is indifferent and cold, a side of medicine that contributes to the suffering and not to the healing, a side of medicine that we should not emulate.

Like Dr. Rabin, I am a physician who has experienced a catastrophic illness prematurely in life, a physician who has become a patient and has experienced an illness from the inside: from the eye of the storm with the eyes of a doctor. I have an illness called the acquired immunodeficiency syndrome (AIDS). I contracted it by an accident with the blood of a patient that I was caring for in 1983. The accident that led to the infection was an ordinary one: A blood-filled capillary tube fractured and cut one of my fingers. The patient was a teenager with leukemia who had been transfused many times. The accident was followed 3 weeks later by an acute febrile illness with cough, sore throat, rash, and lymphadenopathy. At the time, a complete medical evaluation failed to yield a diagnosis, and AIDS was not a consideration because transmission of the human immunodeficiency virus (HIV) through blood at the workplace was unknown. After the acute illness, my feeling of good health returned and for the next 3 years the only reminder I had of the accident was a persistent lymphadenopathy and mild pancytopenia. I went on to complete my residency, became a chief resident, and a fellow in cardiology at the same institution. I married Patricia, a wonderful woman who had just graduated from medical school there. Together we started many projects, pursued many dreams, and had a daughter. Life was going well until December of 1986 when unexplained weight loss led me to see my physician. After a thorough work-up ruled out a malignancy and collagen vascular disease, the recollection of the accident in 1983 led to testing for HIV. My serum, as well as multiple samples of the patient's stored sera, tested positive for HIV. And life changed forever.

Five years have passed since that diagnosis. I remember being so ill at the time that neither my physician nor I thought that I would live long. I follow no magic treatment and know not about cures. But I do know that the efforts to defeat or live with an illness can only succeed if positive attitudes are maintained by both the patient and those caring for the patient. My personal fight against a major illness has been made less difficult by having a fantastic family, a few special friends, and a good physician. Surprisingly, after many years as a physician and several years as a patient, my views of what constitutes a good doctor have become simpler.

A good doctor goes through the struggle of an illness with you, providing support while protecting your dignity and independence, and searches constantly for better options for your care. There is nothing fancy about such qualities; all of us hear about them in our medical training, but many of us forget along the way. So, when I speak about a "good doctor," I do not mean only that technically superior individual who can quote the current literature with ease and recite the different prognoses for illnesses as if they were a memorized telephone book. Much more is needed to care effectively for a patient with a major illness. Much more.

As a patient I have learned that just as important as medical expertise and the proper use of new technologies is the ability of the physician to show legitimate concern, to be there during the bad times, and to provide hope even to the incurable. In the first edition of his *Principles of Internal Medicine,* Tinsley Harrison wrote: "The true physician has a Shakespearean breadth of interest in the wise and the foolish, the proud and the humble, the stoic hero and the whining rogue. He cares for people." In cases without easy answers or for which no effective therapy is available, even the simple feeling on the part of the patient that the physician is doing all that is possible has an important therapeutic effect.

I am fortunate to have a caring physician, one who has been at my side during the worst of times, during the unrelenting fevers and the painful medical procedures and on Saturdays and Sundays, one who has shown a timely presence when an acute event arises. Fortunately for me, my physician believes that grave illnesses are to be tackled aggressively. Maybe his working at a cancer center, caring for patients who often cannot be cured, has imbued him with an aggressive attitude toward treating other grave illnesses like AIDS. I can see how physicians used to treating mostly acute, curable illnesses may become frustrated by AIDS. Sometimes, even my kind and dedicated doctor has nearly lost hope.

Two years ago, for example, I was hospitalized three times within a 2-month period. My blood counts were too low to tolerate the additional drop in leukocytes that the needed medications would cause. We were running out of options for my treatment. I could see in my old friend's eyes that he was feeling defeated. It was my turn to instill in him the "no reason to quit now" attitude. At that moment, it became clearer to me that the relationship between doctor and patient must be a reciprocal one. The doctor gives his or her best in taking care of the patient; the patient, whenever his or her condition allows, must provide feedback and participation in his or her own care, not as a passive recipient of services but rather as a protagonist in the struggle to achieve a better state of health. Teaching patients to be participants in their own care may be as important as teaching them to use insulin or to change diet. The practice of medicine should never be an exercise in domination on the part of the doctor nor a total surrender on the part of the patient.

The good doctor, nurse, or health care worker must not feel the need to demand total submissiveness or to elevate her- or himself to a godly status. And that attitude makes a world of difference for the patient. People with catastrophic illnesses need all the support that can be provided, from everyone who can give it. It does make a difference whether the clerks, nurses, technicians, and doctors are supportive or insulting. Their actions do affect your will to fight, the crucial resolution not to make concessions to the illness. The feeling of being abandoned, that those "caring" for you may not really care, or that they gave up on you long ago, weakens that resolution immensely. The secret to being a good doctor was captured by Dr. Francis Peabody: "The secret of good patient care is to care for the patient." No amount of technology or technical knowledge can substitute for that.

One of the most important dogmas of medicine is "first do not harm." Iatrogenic actions do kill and hurt many patients, but the harm that a physician can do to a patient is not limited to the incorrect use of a medication or invasive procedure. Equally harmful are unwise or inappropriate remarks, especially those that hurt your hope. I will never forget my shock and anger at the response of a physician to a young woman who had AIDS and had been bothered for days with severe headaches. She wanted to know why. The physician responded (while escorting her out of the examining room), "Well you know, this illness is associated with dementia and brain tumors . . . ." Quite a response from somebody who has been given the privilege of caring for others. What that physician had done to the patient's will to fight, to the patient's hope, was nothing less than a radical amputation. Although such thoughtless behavior is not generalized, the apparent indifference born of professional distancing may be.

Being a doctor has not exempted me from feeling the coldness and indifference that medicine can give. I remember clearly when, soon after my diagnosis, my wife and I went to see an "AIDS expert." He sat behind his desk like a businessman discussing the markets, with no show of compassion or even concern for these two colleagues whose lives had just been shattered. He quoted studies and numbers but made no attempt to provide a bit of comfort or hope.

The transition from physician to patient has made me more aware of some aspects of medical care that, although seemingly trivial from the physician's perspective, are terribly important from the patient's perspective. It is what we would call "the little things," like being left waiting indefinitely in the x-ray room, having to wait hours to be seen, being examined with gloves and having my lungs auscultated through a thick sweater, being suddenly looked down on as if I had become something of an inferior nature, only because I became ill. The abuses and mistreatments toward patients that troubled me as a physician now infuriate me as a patient. My protest in that regard is not about receiving special treatment for being a physician; it is simply a call for the basic attention and care that anyone with a major illness should receive. Sometimes we medical people have a terrible tendency to depersonalize the patient, to make him or her a "case." From that moment, he or she is no longer a person with thoughts, dreams, and rights.

A nice man, James D, taught me a lifelong lesson when I was a medical intern. He had come to the hospital for a third opinion regarding a rapidly progressive neurologic illness that had turned him into an emaciated, wheelchair-bound, helpless soul. Because all the consultants had given no hope for cure or improvement, because the multiple complications of his illness required frequent attention, and because of my endlessly busy days as an intern, his care became a bit of a burden. Mr. D had become one more "case." One day his girlfriend gave me a picture of one of his beautiful paintings of wildlife. Later she showed me a picture of Mr. D posing in front of his paintings. Taken only 3 months earlier, it bore no resemblance to the man now lying so ill in bed. He looked so happy, proud, and healthy, like the real person he was. It hit me violently that I had lost sight of my patients as human beings and had begun to see them as a different species: the patient species. I had begun to detach myself from the most important aspect of medicine, and the picture of the recently healthy Mr. D set me back on the right course. I believe that both my patients and I benefited tremendously from that wake-up call. It became one of the most important points in my education and made me question at what point in my training had I begun to separate from the ideas that motivated me to go into medicine.

The process of becoming a doctor is so protracted and arduous that it is easy to forget along the way the initial reasons and ideals for wanting to become a doctor, especially because the current medical curriculum is disease-oriented, not patient-oriented. We need to devote more time and attention to teaching attitudes, skills, and behaviors at the expense of the present preoccupation and fascination with technical knowledge. Because medical school is just the beginning, not the end, of learning to be an effective physician, there is no need to cram ever increasing amounts of information into less time.

Many have questioned whether it is possible to teach concern and compassion to our medical students, because many of one's caring attitudes are imprinted at home and in early schooling. From my experience teaching medical students as a resident, fellow, and chief resident, I feel that students of the 2nd and 3rd year were more receptive to learning attitudes and emulating good bedside manners. By the time the 4th year arrived, those traits appeared to be fading and were being replaced to some extent by cynicism and sarcasm. In most medical schools, the principal teachers and role models for the student are the interns and the residents to whom the students are exposed day and night. When that role model is a tired, overworked person trying to stay afloat, with the best of intentions but with little time for compassion, then the message passed on to the student may be all wrong. It is crucial that when we sit down to refocus medical education, we also address the system of graduate training and improve it so that it will better serve the trainee, his or her patients, and the medical student.

In addition, the selection of those with an active role in teaching students and housestaff must be based on their capacities to be role models and not just on their research merits, ability to draw private patients, or reputation. Often the best role models are not too active in basic research, and the absence of such qualification as a good researcher may handicap their survival in academic medicine. The creation of a separate tenure track for the clinician-teacher would be one way of ensuring that our students and residents profit from their wisdom.

Changing medical education and residency programs, of course, is not easy, but as formidable as such endeavors may seem, devising ways to awaken in the student the good ideals that once motivated him or her to study and practice medicine is paramount. We need to emphasize that the caring function is as vital a part of medical education as the curing function. This need has become even more important with the appearance of AIDS.

For those of you who have a role in the education of younger physicians, it is important that you remember that your attitude in caring for patients with AIDS or any other illness will often be imitated by those you teach. You are the role models whom many of your younger peers will want to imitate. It is not for us to judge the background or preferences of our patients but rather to care for them and to give example to the rest of society.

We, the members of the most humane of professions, must oppose discrimination and bigotry. Discrimination on the basis of an illness is one of the cruelest forms of intolerance that a society can display.

We have seen patients with AIDS get bounced around by a few physicians who, using myriad rationalizations, pretend to justify their refusal to care for these patients. A more subtle form of discrimination, which may be involuntary, is the fatalistic attitude prevalent among some physicians who make therapeutic decisions for patients with AIDS. Granted, AIDS is still incurable, but there are many other incurable illnesses for which physicians and patients do not throw in the towel before giving a formidable fight. Most leukemias and other cancers, cystic fibrosis, rheumatoid arthritis (just to mention a few cruel usurpers of health and happiness), despite being incurable, are treated by physicians in an aggressive manner to give the victims a fighting chance. Why should it be different with AIDS?

Not long ago it was thought that a second episode of *Pneumocystis carinii* pneumonia was reason to give up support. Persons now survive *P. carinii* pneumonia again and again, and this infection can now be prevented. We used to think that there was no way to treat cytomegalovirus infection or to prevent its recurrence. Now there are options for treatment and prevention. Like many other illnesses, AIDS is now a chronic disorder. Knowledge regarding AIDS is constantly increasing and for this reason there should be no room for fatalistic attitudes, from doctors or patients. It is a bad illness, like many others, and like many other illnesses it must be tamed or conquered.

Medicine must lead the way in changing society's fears and misconceptions about AIDS. If medical people show little compassion or discriminate against the victims of this illness, why should the rest of society know or do better?

Five years have passed since my diagnosis, and I have battled multiple complications of this illness. The support and love of my family, my physician, and some friends have given me the strength to put up the best fight I can. They have given me hope. And the fight is worth it; not easy, but worth it, because I have shared with my family the most beautiful of times in the last 5 years. Hope is the one thing that even if we cannot push ourselves as physicians to provide, we should at the very least not deny. To most patients with grave afflictions, hope is the only fuel that keeps them going. I, of course, do not mean that we must provide false assurances to those with major illnesses, but you must let them know that if there is a chance, however small, of a cure or improvement, you will pursue it, and that you will always be on their side searching for those approaches that could make their lives better, looking into that new treatment, or exploring the possible use of that new drug. William Osler advised his peers, "It is not for you to don the black cap and assuming the judicial function, take hope away from any patient . . . ."

I remember from Roni Rabin's book about her father and her family's ordeal with amyotrophic lateral sclerosis that Dr. Rabin from the time of the very first symptoms had a good understanding of what was happening to him, of the incurability of his disease, and of his prognosis. Despite knowing the likely course of his illness, he actively searched for a physician who would support and guide him through a devastating illness. He was no longer searching for cures but for that good physician who would say, "I understand that this illness is happening to *you*, but *we* will face it together." Because it is particularly in cases of catastrophic or incurable illnesses that the role of the physician is more, not less, important, let me suggest that the fewer the therapeutic options available, the greater your involvement with the patient should be. When there is no cure, there is still much to be done to alleviate suffering.

Colleagues, my words have not intended to lecture but rather to invoke. My illness has permitted me to see the worst and the best of people, through the eyes of a physician. Although some awful things have happened to me, I still operate from the premise that humankind is by nature good, that if given the proper stimuli and role models, men and women will rise to their best for the benefit of humanity.

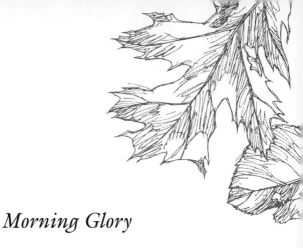

Morning Glory

Your blue petals open
and reflect in them the
splendor of the sky the
brilliance of the sun
on a perfect June morning.

The breeze is light
scented with dogwood
myrtle and honeysuckle;
the symphony of color
and light and air begins.

Your melodious charm
brings me out today
to share your rejoicing
your whispers of thanks
for the glory of this morning.

Martha Harwit, MD

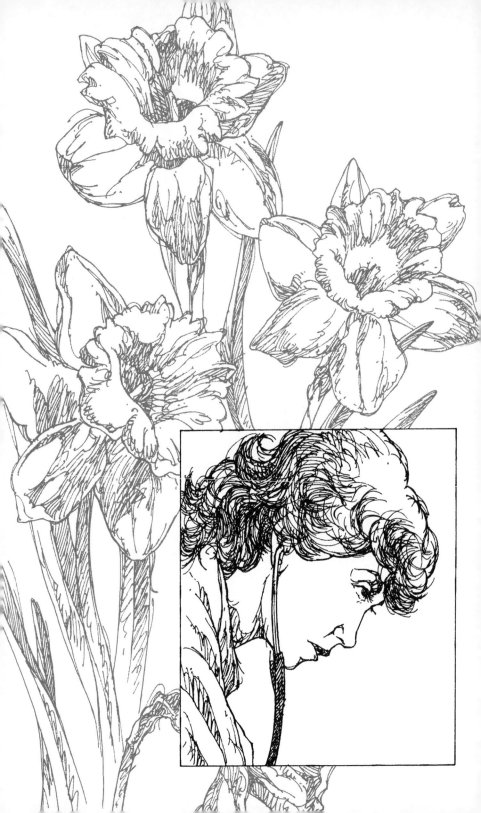

SHE RELATES TO HER PATIENTS

Sonnet XVI

The doctor asked her what she wanted done
With him, that could not lie there many days.
And she was shocked to see how life goes on
Even after death, in irritating ways;
And mused how if he had not died at all
'Twould have been easier—then there need not be
The stiff disorder of a funeral
Everywhere, and the hideous industry,
And crowds of people calling her by name
And questioning her, she'd never seen before,
But only watching by his bed once more
And sitting silent if a knocking came . . .
She said at length, feeling the doctor's eyes,
"I don't know what you do exactly when a person dies."

Edna St. Vincent Millay

Playing God
Michael A. LaCombe, MD

*W*hy she called me first I never figured out. Maybe she had more brains than I gave her credit for. All she had said was, My husband has passed away, Doctor. Can you come over?

That was it: flat monotone, no emotion, just matter-of-fact. Now I'm one of those old-fashioned doctors who still makes house calls on certain occasions, and this was definitely one of those occasions. I could feel it in the pit of my stomach. I grabbed my clothes, got dressed in the bathroom so as not to wake my wife, brushed the snow from the car, and headed over to their farm. A storm had passed through unannounced, leaving snow everywhere. It was the kind of night where, once you get out into it, you're glad you're there—everything blanketed in rolling white, not a rift in the cover—so cold and clear the stars hang down out of the sky just above the snow. On a night like that, you had trouble believing there could be any evil in the world.

From the bend in the road I could see the light from their kitchen far off, sparkling down the crystals of snow. I pulled the car in at the barest suggestion of a driveway, turned off the motor, and pushed through the drifts up to the porch. I let myself in. The house was quiet as a tomb. The kitchen clock gave off a quiet hum. On the face of the refrigerator were plastered the kids' school papers: spelling tests and arithmetic, maps colored in Crayola, and the minimal artwork of the early grades. There was a "Mom-Dad-and-Me" family portrait—"Mom" about a quarter the size of "Dad," who occupied center stage, and "Me" off to the side, a stick figure without arms—no mouth drawn in. I stepped through the kitchen and found Kitty sitting in the darkened living room in a straight-backed chair, staring off, trance-like, in shock maybe. What appeared to be small marbles lay scattered on the carpet. I picked one up. It was a pearl.

"Where's Earl?" I asked her.

"In the bedroom?" said Kitty. She always said everything as though it were a question. She motioned with her head.

"Where are the kids?"

"At my sister's?" she answered.

"You all right?" I asked.

She nodded.

I took a deep breath and headed into the bedroom, expecting the worst. I wasn't disappointed. Earl lay flat on the bed, a bullet hole above his right ear. The left half of his cranium and its contents were splattered next to him on the bedroom wall. I began to run a cold sweat. Even after all the years of small-town practice, being called in for mangled bodies and auto wrecks, botched amateur abortions, deceased elderly pensioners not found for days, and—worst of all—the abused children—that, worst of all—despite all of that hardening up, a scene like this still could weaken you at the knees. I swallowed against the sweat, looked away, looked back again, and had to look away. It was hard to stay clinical. Doctors have trouble with violent death. Disease we learn to accept. But not this.

I surveyed the scene. Earl's .30-.30 Winchester lay on the floor just inside the door. A half-empty bottle of Schenley's stood next to the bed, within easy reach. Earl lay on the bed fully dressed, shoes on, with that eternal gaze that can make your skin crawl.

The rest of the room was precise and neat. The top of the bureau was uncluttered: a brush, a comb, a mirror, all arranged just so, and an ash tray full of change. A wedding picture of Kitty and Earl stood off to the side. The bedside table held a small reading lamp, the shade a shocking white against the dark streaks of Earl's blood on the wall. There was a Bible and an old clothbound book, its title faded, and a pair of woman's reading glasses folded on top. There were no clothes lying about. The closet doors were closed. The window drapes hung just so. All this tidiness framing the mess of Earl's body.

I went back out to the living room to Kitty. She hadn't moved a muscle, except that her eyes had the look of a cornered mouse.

"What happened?" I asked her.

"He shot himself?" Kitty answered.

"Shot himself," I said.

She nodded.

"Kitty . . ." my voice trailed off. I sat down in a chair opposite her and looked at her for a long minute.

"Kitty, we go way back don't we?"

She nodded again.

Some 30 years ago I had brought her into this world, supported her through her mother's premature death, and 20 years later, delivered babies of her own. I had seen her boy through a bad case of spinal meningitis, and harped at her father's cigarette smoking, in the end burying him because of it.

But, through the most of it there had been Kitty. She held the record for most abused woman in Taylor County. There had been the time I had hospitalized her for a hairline fracture of the mandibular ramus, a both-bones fracture of the left forearm, and God knows how many internal injuries, for the better part of a week. We had Earl all wrapped up and ready to send down to the state prison. And then Kitty wouldn't sign the papers. The night I hospitalized her from that episode I stopped by her father's house just to check on things. Al was in a murderous rage. I could hardly blame him.

"I'm going to kill the son of a bitch. I'm going to kill the son of a bitch," was all he kept muttering. He'd look at me with his reddened, burning eyes, and I knew he meant it.

"Al," I said, "you do that and you'll wind up in prison yourself."

"I don't give a damn," he said.

"And Earl will get off."

"Earl will be dead," he answered.

"And your grandchildren will hate you for the rest of their lives," I said, "for killing their father."

At that, the hardness left him and he gave it up.

"I'm going to tell you something else, Al," I said. "In 2 weeks Kitty will be right back with him and there isn't a damn thing you can do about it."

Soon Kitty did go back with Earl. You had trouble saying whose sickness was worse. But there was no question about Kitty's suffering. Or her father's. It was the same scenario for some 10 years, Kitty coming into the emergency room, badly beaten, meekly asking to see me, Al flying into a rage, and, in the early years, loading up his gun, resolving to put Earl away, later resigning himself to this terrible disease that both Earl and Kitty were torturing him with. Two other times Kitty had been so severely beaten that she required hospitalization. Each time we got the town police involved, had Earl arrested, had the complaint papers all filled out. All sealed, and delivered, except that Kitty would never sign the papers. And she always went back to him.

"You know, Doc," said the Chief of Police one day, "some day one of these two is going to wind up dead."

Kitty shifted in her chair and brought me back to the darkened living room. I turned to look at her. I was her doctor, her family's doctor. She'd level with me.

"What really happened?" I asked her.

"I heard the gun go off?" she said. "I went in. And he was dead."

"I didn't see a suicide note, Kitty," I said, pressing her. "Did he leave a note? People usually leave a note in these situations."

"No," she said. "There wasn't any note." Her voice fell. As tentative as she was, Kitty wouldn't budge. I thought later, looking back on it, that this was probably the first time in her life she had made up her mind and stuck to it.

"Kitty . . . ." I didn't know what else to say to her. She shifted nervously in the chair and I saw her wince. She held her left arm close to her body.

There she was, Al's little girl—everybody's little girl. I could remember Kitty skipping into my office at 5 full of happiness and life, for her preschool shots, and coming in again at 12, the apple of her daddy's eye, for her camp physical. We were there, Al and I, on that crisp November day when Kitty bagged her first deer. And I sat at the head table, at her wedding reception—she and Earl the handsome couple—Kitty proudly wearing her mother's string of pearls that Al had surprised her with on that day. And after that all those hospital admissions . . . Kitty . . . most abused woman in the whole county.

But there was a lot more that went into this case. There had been Leon Tilley's murder 2 years before. He had been found dead in his hay field, two bullet holes at the base of his skull, relieved of a large amount of cash. For a year nothing happened. Tilley had been one popular old man, the kind of Norman Rockwell farmer everybody stops to talk to, wisdom written all over his face. The town was pretty unhappy with what they saw as police inaction. Then four teenagers and a drug dealer were apprehended and the papers were filled with yellow journalism for 6 months: stories of bad cops, barflies, drugs, and witnesses who lied. The kind of stuff that's not supposed to happen in the country. The whole county salivated. After all the publicity, the big-city lawyers, and backroom deals, the D.A. managed only one conviction. Now everybody was still screaming for the police chief's head and small-time entrepreneurs were getting rich selling T-shirts that read:

Come to Herkimer and get away with murder.

I looked at Kitty, and then into the bedroom, then back at Kitty again. I nodded to myself. Yes indeed, I thought, the Chief would dearly love to get his hands on this one. He needed this one.

One time back along, I had a bad baby on my hands, a newborn with hydrocephalus and a big cyst at the base of the neck—the crippled-for-life kind of baby you see once in a lifetime. I watched that baby struggle and watched and didn't do a damn thing to save it and apologized to the family afterwards, explaining it was a stillborn, lying to them. That was the one time I played God and it aggravated me, I can tell you. I went home that night and yelled at my wife, kicked the dog, and drank too much—brooded for weeks and never talked about it. It can eat at you. There had never been a second time until Kitty.

I grabbed one of the kitchen chairs and a dish towel and went back into the bedroom. In a few minutes I was on the phone and had the dispatcher get hold of the Chief. Shortly he was at the other end of the line, sleepy, gruff, trying to be important.

"Chief," I said, "I'm at Earl Staples' house. He's finally done himself in. He got drunk and shot himself with his deer rifle . . . yeah, I'm at the house now . . . well, it looks to me like he rested the gun on a chair next to the bed, and then lay himself down and shot himself in the temple. Clear suicide in my book. I'll be signing it out that way . . . Yeah, she's here with me. I'll drive her over to her sister's. I'd sure appreciate it if you'd send one of your men over here to clean things up . . . . Thanks Chief."

I put the phone down and turned back to Kitty. She was staring at the floor. She hadn't moved. I sighed, slapped my thighs, and got up to go.

"Where's your coat, Kitty? I'll drive you over to Kate's, and in the morning," I said, nodding to her left arm, "you come over to the office so I can set that fracture for you one last time."

Her Daughter in My Office
Andrew N. Wilner, MD

*H*ow plump she was, thick with that extra chromosome! Such large eyes made me wonder was it really true? And coffee-colored skin I had never seen before in a Down patient. So astute she was, pointing knowingly to my diploma! So smart, this child of 33, or did I expect so little? Her smile engaged me and for a second I forgot her problem. So loving she was! Could I be sure she was an accident? Or by chance conceived too late? Her aging mother's unfortunate gift, yet the two of them together seemed natural, as if it were meant to be. "Seizures Doctor everyday, I don't know what to do. She's a good girl, takes her medicines, why don't they work Doctor? She falls, drops like a stone. Wait, you'll see."

True, every medicine tried, therapeutic levels without result. My mind focused on her thick chart to hide, I think, from this reality. What could I do? I had no tools. I could not change the genes. Then, an incredible crash! Her skull against the wall, an inhuman thud. "Yes, Doctor, like that. She drops"

"Oh, I see."

I see, my God, she's not kidding! My face pale, a doctor responded.

"Yes, well, glad to witness that. Now we know what we're talking about. Perhaps some fancy surgery, the epilepsy kind they're talking about. Let's think about it."

"Thank you, Doctor, so much." They left, her daughter now more wobbly after this spell.

"One moment please!" Desperate I reach out to give a prescription.

"In the meantime, before the miracles, a helmet might do nicely."

Motke

Joseph Herman, MD

$\mathcal{M}$ost of us have at least one candidate for "my most unforget-table patient"; the more fortunate may even have several. Mine is Motke and I am not sure if it would have been any easier to forget him had I not been his doctor. He was one of those people who embody a whole way of being; he stood over and against the materialistic, communal idealism of those among whom he lived. There was an air of saintliness about him but he would have laughed at the description, for he was an agnostic. He walked with a limp from childhood polio. The defect made him unfit for the occupations involving sword or ploughshare through which men established themselves as useful members of kibbutz society.

When a doctor feels affection for his patient, the outcome of any interaction between them may be improved. There was no way not to show warmth to Motke, but I do not flatter myself that what must have been obvious to him in all our dealings had anything to do with the surprisingly long time this story covers. By way of more explicit and clinical introduction, let it be said that he was destined to outlive some of his coronary arteries and most of his myocardium by a score of years.

My first encounter with Motke took place in 1965 when I was an intern in the department of medicine at a 300-bed peripheral hospital in the Jezreel Valley. He lay there with a great shock of white hair spread around his delicate features, a veritable halo of dishevelment, looking unwell but resigned to his circumstances. One of the senior physicians—we were making rounds—showed me his cardiogram with its towering QRS complexes, its giant T-waves, and its S-T segments depressed 5 mm or more below baseline. It had, of course, been taken at rest and eloquently expressed the chest pain for which he had been admitted. Although nothing more than a streamer of slick paper, checkered gray and black, the cardiogram appeared to me a death warrant. After rounds, the senior physician told me to do an admission history and physical examination on Motke and, as if to warn me not to draw too close emotionally, added that he thought the patient was not long for this world.

Motke and I hit it off quite well, perhaps because I was a full decade older than most of the other junior staff members and had spent 9 years farming. I have no recollection of the anamnestic details he gave in reply to my questions. I do remember his thin, wiry physique and the heaving ventricle, not only palpable but also visible. The point of maximum impulse, too, showed how far it could wander from its appointed place when things went wrong.

Somehow, Motke made it through the week and was discharged home to his kibbutz in the Beisan Valley, 25 miles away, with a diagnosis of coronary artery disease. I learned that he was a horticulturist with an international reputation who specialized in growing rose bushes. Letters asking for advice were delivered from all over the world to his room, which resembled a monk's cell. The duties of an intern made me forget him and we did not meet again until nearly 4 years had passed.

When my residency was completed, I looked for suitable work in ambulatory medicine. The health maintenance organization that insured almost all of the denizens of the Jezreel and Beisan Valleys and also ran the regional hospital assigned me to five border settlements, one of which was Motke's home. After a quarter of a century of backbreaking labor by its pioneers, who withstood unimaginable hardships, the area was now quite green. It lay some 700 feet below sea level, and noontime summer temperatures hovered around 40 °C but had been known to climb as high as 53 °C. It was under intermittent mortar and small arms fire from across the Jordan River, and military prowess and resourcefulness in repairing damaged machinery were more in demand than expertise in horticulture. In particular, there was no money in rose bushes and younger members of Motke's kibbutz cast an envious eye on the little parcel of land, just inside the perimeter fence, where his nursery was located.

It took some time for me to adjust to the prevailing, war-like atmosphere that was to persist for 2 years. I am afraid that during those heroic days I had a tendency to regard wounds from shell fragments as the only significant medical condition and to look down on patients who were troubled over trivial complaints. I certainly wasn't much good at eliciting their concerns beyond the occasional confession of feeling uptight because of "the situation." However, for Motke I always had time, possibly because I could really do so little for him and because he stood out as unique and refined in comparison with the rough-and-ready surroundings. He came to the clinic infrequently and on each occasion it turned out that he had stopped taking the pills I had so optimistically prescribed on his previous visit. Beta-blockers were now available but Motke didn't like being medicated, although he was far too tactful to reveal this to me. He seemed to know the secret of living without health at a safe distance from medicine. He believed that disease and death are part of life, which goes on without regard to quality. I often felt that with some knowledge of homeopathy or nature cures I could have done him far more good.

Motke spoke an elegant although somewhat archaic Hebrew, quoting freely from Scripture not out of belief but because he liked a well-turned phrase. I am surprised today that I know nothing of his origins in Poland. He seemed faintly anachronistic, yet so much a part of the present that it was difficult to connect him with siblings or parents. He was definitely not happy; the kibbutz had reached a stage when family life was becoming ever more central. A confirmed bachelor, he radiated a certain inner peace despite spending most of every 24 hours alone. He withstood all blandishments to retire honorably and surrender his few acres to something more profitable. Every year, with several of the young women, he would put on a floral show in the spacious hall where cultural activities usually took place. Dozens of varieties of roses were then on display and people came from the neighboring settlements to a defiant demonstration of the beautiful and the transient, briefly preserved from an environment that seemed hostile in every way. Many volunteers passed through the kibbutz in those days, looking for a taste of communal life and the occasional surge of adrenalin that the odd mortar shell could provide. Over the years, I would meet one or another of them, always hearing that the most memorable aspect of his or her kibbutz experience was being assigned for a day to work in Motke's nursery.

One morning I awoke to the realization that I had been working in the Beisan Valley for 17 years! My wife and I took stock, and, since our nest was on the verge of emptying, decided we should move on. Perhaps, too, we feared the day when I would have to attend to the last illnesses of people to whom we were bound by ties of a shared fate and similar ideals. Once a year thereafter a New Year's card would arrive from Motke, but we never saw him again. We heard later that, some 20 years after my first encounter with him, he was found dead between the rows of his beloved rose bushes with a peaceful look on his face. He had exceeded the three-score and ten allotted us by the ninetieth Psalm and even outlived the average Israeli male.

When I wondered what impelled me to write of him at this particular time, two answers suggested themselves. The first has to do with one of Jerusalem's loveliest parks that I happened into just a few days ago. It comprises lawns, trees, a small lake, and a network of moats spanned here and there by a rustic bridge, along with thousands of rose bushes about to flower. Two or three of the varieties Motke perfected grow there, identified by little metal signs.

The second answer is concerned with the term "modern medicine." When Motke was admitted to the hospital 27 years ago, we believed fervently that our practice was current and that our patients were benefiting from the best the profession could offer. Indeed, in historical perspective 1965 definitely belongs to the modern era. In the very shadow of Mt. Gilboa where, three millennia earlier Saul and Jonathan had perished, the department of medicine had just received a Lown DC cardioverter. Various antibiotics were available, as were powerful new diuretics and hypotensive agents. Our general surgeons were doing splenorenal shunts for portal hypertension and sophisticated workups for Hirschprung disease. We read the latest journals avidly, knowing that it would take a few years until the dazzling new technologies reported there reached us, but feeling that they were already within our grasp. As always, the advances were uneven rather than across the entire front, and I mention some of the measures we took against ischemic heart disease with a sense of embarrassment because they now seem hopelessly crude. We used nitrates, still standbys for angina pectoris, with no appreciation of tolerance. We administered dipyridamole because even 5 years later a respected textbook said it might improve collateral circulation. We prescribed monoamine oxidase inhibitors believing that, in addition to their sedative influence, they might have some direct effect on the ischemic myocardium. Finally, we gave propylthiouracil for intractable angina in the hope that the hypothyroid state would make fewer metabolic demands on the heart.

Could we have done more for Motke had all that is written here happened two decades later? Could we have added years to life, or life to years as the saying goes? Would he have allowed us angiography, percutaneous transluminal coronary angioplasty, bypass, or transplantation? I seriously doubt it. Imperfect from childhood, he did not pursue any ideal of health, nor could longevity, in and for itself, ever have been a good in his eyes. He wrested a score of summers from the absurd, confronting it clear-eyed but with some bemusement and, when it was enough, he simply let go.

Veiled Purpose

These many years the vision and the words
keep creeping back to slyly haunt and mock
in me the Healing Art so poorly used,
a beamless beacon with no light to rouse
to view John's darkly shadowed mind, and sense
its nest of hopeless phantoms urging death.

I thought it hard to say to him straight out
"there's cancer there," and leave no shred of hope,
but chose instead to pantomime the truth
with mealy words to soften what they meant.
But while I strove to shield him from the hurt,
he coolly saw the truth and laid his plan.

And though again and yet again, as if
he did not know, but must have surely known,
he prompted me to frankly speak about
his ill though dire, and not to doubt that he
could boldly and with utter braveness face
whatever fate decreed and I advised,

I'd say "there is a lesion in your lung
that might become malign" but there was this
to do and that and never answer straight.
He too, much like a lawyer at the bar,
would harass, beg, and cutely fake his case
and wear me down and make me doubt myself.

And so at last, as not before or since,
I was not circumspect but said it straight,
that "Yes, you have a cancer in the lung,"
which verified his darkest thought, and gave
the sign that set his deadly goblins free
to machinate his suicidal bent.

The next day came and with it my reward,
John's daughter called to tell me he was dead
and wonder what I'd said to him the day
before that made him seek relief by gas.
I grieved, and told her what we both had said,
but then her silence seemed to scream my guilt.

It may be that she had no wish to hurt,
but when she asked no more I lost my chance
to plead "he coaxed unvarnished truth from me,"
and challenge that she never came or called
to warn about her father's troubled thoughts,
and share the pending legacy of guilt.

In retrospect he left a triple cloud:
She, sadly failed to sense his will to die,
I, failed to solve his urgent quest for truth,
He, schemed and made me party to his plan:
My words to validate his deadly act,
to toll his end and sire my remorse.

Alfred P. Ingegno, MD

No Time for Flowers
Anne Scheetz, MD

The doctor's late now and that means she'll be mad. She hasn't called either, like she usually does when she's held up at the hospital and she'll be 5 minutes late getting to the office. Only now it's going to be at least 10 minutes. That means she's stuck in traffic so she'll be mad she's late and mad at the traffic. She plans her days so all the driving is easy and she doesn't hit any of the busy times. She says her time is valuable and so is her patients' time, and she owes them the respect of giving them the time they're scheduled for. I'm amazed how she can get in and out of those rooms right on time and, if the day's going well and she's happy, she never acts in a hurry. When she's mad because she has to hurry, it's different; she might try to hide it, but I can tell, and nothing goes as smoothly. She can't help getting mad when some idiot pages her for something she says a child could have solved or when there's an accident that she says could have been avoided with a modicum of competence. (I'm pretty sure she called it a modicum.)

My mother got me this job for the summer, working part time as a receptionist because Dr. Shaw's regulars all take turns going on vacation. It seems to be okay for a guy to answer the phone and meet people when they come in. All the other people who do this are girls, but nobody seems to mind me being a guy, not the patients or the girls, and certainly not my Mom. She says since I'm thinking of being a doctor this is a good way to find out what goes on in a doctor's office without having to know anything except how to be polite. I get to hear a lot from the patients and the staff, and sometimes the nurse asks me to come back and help her with something, like getting an old lady out of a wheelchair or holding down a kid who has to get his blood drawn or, if it's not real busy, she might show me something, like how to do an EKG.

One thing I'd like about being a doctor, I could afford nice clothes and get to drive a sharp car like Dr. Shaw's. I'd like to be able to tell people what's good for them and what to do to take care of themselves and sound like there's no way I could be wrong. I'd like to have people say to me, "Oh, thank you, Doctor, you've helped me so much." I'd like to see them smile and look like they feel good when they leave, even though they came in looking miserable. I'd like to have people brag about me, saying how smart their doctor is and how handsome (only they call Dr. Shaw pretty, and they say how nice it is to see a doctor who knows how to look good). I'd like to hear them tell each other what I said about this new drug they're advertising on TV and say that I saved somebody's life by putting him in the hospital in the nick of time after the other doctor just kept seeing him in the office.

There are a bunch of old—older, I'm supposed to say—people sitting in the waiting room. Some are patients—they're here to see the doctor—but lots of them are husbands and wives or just friends, or they're here to get medicine from the pharmacy. They like to sit and talk. They've all lived in this neighborhood their whole lives so they all know each other. They give each other rides and go out for coffee together on their way home. They don't notice whether the doctor's on time or a little late, and Mary Jo—she's Dr. Shaw's nurse—is real good at making sure nobody realizes they're waiting. She takes them back just a few minutes late, and takes her time weighing them, and asks about their married daughters and their grandchildren, and asks to go over their medicine bottles. Sometimes I help, too—like I'll ask them if I have the right phone number for the person to contact in case of an emergency. The patients don't mind so much her being late, but Dr. Shaw does.

Anyway, now I can hear her in the back, just a couple of words, because she's 12 minutes late and won't waste time this morning saying hello and asking how everybody's doing. I still go stick my head through the window to say, "Good morning, Dr. Shaw," and she says, "Good morning," back. She's polite—she would be—but it's not the same as when she's in a good mood. She's in a rush so she doesn't smile and hardly even looks at me and her face is stern and worried-looking. I brought in some flowers this morning—the kind my Mom likes—yellow and white ones. I brought them for the whole office, not just for Dr. Shaw, but I know she likes them; she always stops to look at flowers and smell them. Now I know she won't notice them until maybe the end of the day—she won't even come out here now until all the patients are gone. I hope they still look nice by the time she gets to see them. Maybe when she finally looks at them she'll smile and not look worried anymore.

A Magnificent Whole

John T. Lynn III, MD

I introduced myself, and a touchy silence filled the room. Motorcycle people, I thought, glancing at the patient and his two visitors. My stethoscope felt sticky as I turned to find a chair.

With the chart resting on my crossed legs, I asked, "What problem are you having, Mr. Hugo?"

The woman on the other side of the bed replied, "He has a bleeding ulcer, but his left knee and foot are what really hurt." Her voice was staccato, yet strangely monotonal. She faced the head of the bed, her profile partly covered by tarry hair. After answering my question, her head drifted backward like a turtle withdrawing into its shell, causing the pale skin beneath her chin to bulge. The crumbled words on her snug black T-shirt advised: "Experience is what you get when you don't get what you want."

I turned to Mr. Hugo. "How long has your leg hurt?"

The woman replied, "Since he came to the hospital, beginning of the week."

Mr. Hugo was staring at the opposite wall. Strings of hair, the color of used dishwater, fell over his ears, just touching the beard that grew from his face and neck. His beard parted widely in the shape of a smile, showing a dark space bordered by chipped teeth. The blueness of his eyes seemed muted, like a midmorning ocean sky.

"Do you see anything at all?" I asked.

He laughed, his large abdomen shaking the bedsheets. "Not a thing," he bellowed.

Again I focused on his leg pain, and the woman answered each question. Her gaze wandered over my head and slightly to the right; my eyes swept the floor. Frustration yielded to curiosity and I asked, "What relation are you to Mr. Hugo?"

"We've been engaged for years. We can't get married. We'd lose half our money," she said.

I asked Mr. Hugo to show me where he hurt. His fiancée nimbly slid her hand between the bars of the siderail and, with a lover's touch, slowly skimmed her fingers along his thigh until she found the swollen warm knee. When I gently touched his knee, he sharply rolled his leg away in pain.

Mr. Hugo's sudden movement startled the other visitor, a barrel of a man with curly hair who had been sitting silently at the foot of the bed. My eyes and mouth gaped. He had at least 20 earrings hanging from his head!

I tried to resume the examination but kept turning toward the earring man. Finally I said, "Excuse me, sir, but I have to take a closer look."

Mr. Hugo and his fiancée grinned. The earring man seemed bewildered by my attention. I inspected the turquoise and emerald-like stones dangling from his ears, the silver crosses and stars hanging from his lips and cheeks. He sighed, and the diamonds anchored to his nose twinkled in the room's white light.

Amazed I asked, "Do these get infected—do you have earrings on the other parts of your body?" He studied my lips and had the bemused expression of a portly geology professor returning from an unusually successful rock collecting trip.

Mr. Hugo called, "It's not like a rash, Doc!"

His fiancée giggled. "Must be a sight."

"Does this jewelry have any religious significance?" I asked.

"If he were that religious, he wouldn't be our friend," Mr. Hugo roared. "He adds one piece of jewelry every year."

"Where do you people come from?" I asked, imagining the answer might be The Land of Oz, or even Los Angeles.

"South Colorado Springs," the woman answered matter-of-factly.

"Where did you meet?"

"Years ago, we were students together at the Colorado School for the Deaf and the Blind. We kind of take care of each other," she said; then she and Mr. Hugo began to laugh deeply. Seeing his friends laugh, the earring man chortled, setting his jewelry in chaotic motion.

Yes, I thought, together they make one—a magnificent whole—she with her keen ear, maternal concern, and sensitive touch; Mr. Hugo battling suffering with unbridled laughter; and the earring man with his sight and artistic sense. Three people—bonded by trust, need, and experience.

Looking at them I explained, "A part of you has gout. I can treat that. I think you'll all feel more comfortable."

Frame and Focus
Norman R. Epstein, MD

*P*eriodically she comes to my office with her husband. I can count on Betty coming in promptly, docile spouse in tow, each time there is a change in habit, an obvious ailment, or just a feeling that something is wrong. Ravaged by Alzheimer disease, he smiles easily at any and all instructions, although getting him to stand is a trick and using the exam table is almost impossible.

She is infinitely patient, as she would have to be, explaining her concerns and observations, reaffirming her willingness to live for two people most of every day while he stares around the room uncomprehending. Somehow, we always manage to get him examined. His overall physical health is remarkably solid—heart, lungs, kidneys, and bowels aren't even close to significant decline, and his medical problems have been minor and easily handled.

Usually there is enough extra time to talk with Betty about herself and how she's managing. Although the conversation is an opportunity for her to voice her needs and concerns for the future, we don't dwell on this because she shows no change in her willingness to care for him, despite the fact that she is over 70 years old. Often we digress and speak of travel, because we both enjoy this. She and her husband traveled widely before, and she kept extensive diaries. On this particular day, she reflects about their last trip together, to China for a full month. "It was the first time I had to admit that something was wrong," she said. "He remembered just one of the 28 hotels we stayed at."

On their return, the medical workup began, with the diagnosis of Alzheimer disease quickly suspected and confirmed in time by his rapid and steady progression down that mysterious trail where the logic of the world fades and then disappears forever. Now he spends his days diapered and dressed, sitting and looking out the window, at TV or just with his own indecipherable thoughts, smiling and waiting for the next action to be brought to him.

"He was a wonderful photographer," she continued. "I was a writer, but he was always able to see things in a special way. Able to capture the essence of a place in a way I never could." She looks at him fondly. I wonder how close to her patience and forbearance I could possibly come were I in her role, and I have my doubts. And if I were in his role? Too frightening, yet possible—why not? What deep wells would I swim in and how would I be cared for? Who would do it? Where? I dare not think too long on this.

"You know," she says, "it's strange, but I believe the best photographs of all he's taken were done on that trip to China. He seemed to see more profoundly than ever before. They were his best . . . but his last."

We part with wishes for good health and a radiant smile from her.

Perhaps I'll firm up those plans for a family trip to Oaxaca this year—there are so many places on our "wish list" to see, and time seems more fragile than ever after a visit from a patient like this. Of course, I'll bring my camera. I always do. I hope I can capture the feel of the place, get those elusive great pictures—but what will I think if my photographs are unusually good, uncommonly perceptive, a bit beyond what I have ever done before?

Adrienne

Dennis H. Novack, MD

I met Adrienne as an intern, when I admitted her to the hospital. She was an attractive, engaging woman, a junior faculty member at a nearby liberal arts college. She spoke with an Australian accent in a low voice that was serious, earnest, and playful all at once. She had done some camping a few weeks before and strained her back. She was sure that carrying heavy packs had caused the strain, but since it hadn't gotten any better, her physician felt that she should come into the hospital.

I guess I wasn't a very good interviewer back then. Somehow I had failed to elicit the fact that she had a mastectomy.

I was still at a stage when I felt uneasy examining young women. When it was time for the breast exam, I raised her gown to below her ribs and hesitantly began to examine her breasts. I was shocked that her left breast was missing. "Oh that," she responded cheerfully, "I had cancer a few years ago but the mastectomy cured it. I don't give it much thought anymore." I was instantly saddened, knowing that the cause of her back pain might be a metastatic lesion. I stumbled through the rest of our conversation. I agreed with her that the heavy pack had probably caused her back strain and that with a little conservative care, she would be better in no time.

The following afternoon I looked at her spine films with my resident. I remember him saying, "She's got it, all right. She'll need to be checked for other mets. She'll need castration, radiation, chemo, the works." I didn't go back to see her. She was a private patient, after all, and I was superfluous to her care. Besides, I couldn't face her. I knew she would ask me about her prognosis. I knew she would be afraid of death. I couldn't talk to her about it. So I spent the next couple of days being angry with myself for not going back and talking to people about how you talk to patients with metastatic cancer. Finally one of my psychiatric colleagues gave me the best advice.

"Why don't you just go in and say, 'Hello'?"

"Damn," I thought, "he's right," and went up to her room. She had been discharged.

I didn't see Adrienne again for about 6 or 8 months. Then, her oncologist approached me.

"Do you remember Adrienne S?" she asked. "She has quite a lot of feelings about what it's like to have cancer and is very articulate. She wants to speak to a small group of physicians to help them understand how to better care for their patients with cancer." I said that I would be glad to organize such a conference and called Adrienne, arranging to meet her for lunch.

That lunch was extraordinary. We spent a couple of hours talking, about her experiences mostly. I felt moved and told her that her insights and feelings were too precious to share with only a few physicians. She agreed to be part of a panel discussion that also included her oncologist, a nurse, a minister, and me. I advertised it for all hospital personnel.

About 200 people attended. There was a good deal of anger in Adrienne's initial remarks, mostly about physicians' lack of empathy and avoidance of her and about the hospital's lack of attention to the little things. (For example, she couldn't wash her hair in the hospital and, for a woman who cared about her appearance, she found this degrading.) She talked about what the cancer had done to her and for her, about her feelings of disconnectedness from her past and from normal life. She talked about how hospital personnel simply called her "Adrienne" without asking how she preferred to be addressed. She talked with appreciation about the student nurse who had naively inquired about her life. She spoke about her prognosis. Clearly her oncologist's honesty and respect had helped her cope. "What a remarkable woman," a friend said later. "It's hard to understand how people believe there is a just and merciful God out there. If there were, how could He let a woman like this die?"

I saw Adrienne often after that. My wife and I had dinner with her; I met her for lunch a couple of times; but mostly I saw her during her repeated admissions to the hospital.

I remember one Saturday, when I was on call and having a slow night. I had been feeling sad about Adrienne's increasing disability. Around 9 p.m., I brought my guitar up to her room. She was sharing the room with another young woman about her age who I had cared for when she was in the ICU. Karen had been septic and quite sick but was now on the mend. I remember thinking about the contrast between the two young women, one getting better and one getting worse. I played my guitar and we all sang folk songs. Adrienne sang all of the lyrics to "On Top of Old Smokey." I had never actually heard all of the verses before or realized until then that it was the song of a jilted lover. It has been hard for me to sing that song ever since. As I left to go, Adrienne called me over and gave me a friendly kiss.

On another occasion I passed by her room around midnight and saw that she was awake. I walked in and sat and talked with her for awhile. Adrienne spoke with me about her former husband. Not wanting to take care of an invalid, he had left her after her cancer was diagnosed. We talked about her social life, which had been pretty drab recently. I remember her comment: "Doctors don't pay attention to your real needs." We sat in silence after that and then changed the subject.

Inevitably her cancer spread to her brain. She had trouble walking. I had lunch with her one day before she went to radiation therapy. Adrienne was infuriated with her Dean who had canceled her teaching for that semester. She was too weak to go to class but not too weak to hold class in her apartment, which she had fully intended to do. "Damn it. I'm alive until I die," she said, and had resumed teaching.

On another occasion, I asked her why she cared for me, as she had been recently telling me. I felt I hadn't really done anything for her. She told me she cared for me not for what I was able to do but for who I was. "But," I thought, "isn't who you are assessed by what you do?" Still, I was touched that she cared for me and felt I had made a difference in her life.

Near the end of my residency, she was admitted just as I was leaving for a vacation. I went up to see her before I left and stood beside her while her sister, who had flown in from Australia, sat by. I held her hand and talked with her a bit. She was now somewhat confused. She talked in medical terms about her disease and I remember saying sadly, "So many words you have had to learn." I wanted to tell her I loved her, and kiss her goodbye, but I didn't, not wanting to admit to her, and myself, that she was dying. I left for the sun. When I came back, Adrienne was gone, her body shipped back to Australia, the memorial service days earlier. I had missed it all.

Adrienne was the first—and the last—patient to become my friend, although a number of patients have called me "friend" since. I never again became so emotionally involved with a patient but, in the end, I was grateful for the experience. Adrienne deepened my understanding of patients' experiences of terminal illness and helped me overcome my fears of relating to these patients. She also made me aware of the potential for love between doctors and patients: What are the meanings and implications of attraction and caring between doctor and patient? How do clinicians work out the conflicting emotions that sometimes arise?

Michael

Barely fifteen,
Played center for your team,
Small town Georgia.

Marrow transplantation,
Matched sister, older than you,
A gift of life, possibly.

Nine hundred rads, whole body,
Death certain
Without your sister's gift.

A race with death
Those twenty-five days;
Lost.

G. Nicholas Rogentine, Jr., MD

The Chicken Man

Shelley Jones, MD

$\mathcal{H}$e came down off the mountain with chest pain and an aching in his gums. It had been years since his last trip to town. That was when his sister had the shingles on her leg and couldn't stand to drive the truck. He wouldn't have gone then, except they had run out of chicken feed. Today, when his color turned pale and he told Buena he thought he might die, she insisted she bring him to the doctor.

He sat on the passenger's side cradling his left arm as if it were broken. As they turned from the rutted road onto the smooth pavement, he felt as if he were going to vomit, as if he were on a roller coaster. The trees grew up over the road and made a cool tunnel, but later, when the trees thinned out, the open fields stifled him. The sunlight made him sweat. The town reached toward the foot of the mountain, from where they had come. Smells from burger restaurants made his mouth ache more, and he vomited into a rusty coffee can that Buena had brought along for such an emergency.

He walked into the waiting room rubbing his left arm. Sweat was pouring down his bare back, soaking his overalls. He was hunched over, with his Adam's apple stuck out and his neck bent like a turkey buzzard. His hair was butched. His teeth were gone except for a few tobacco-stained stubs. He wore a pair of muddy cowboy boots. He felt the people eyeing him, felt their stares pressing in on his chest. He was glad when the nurse took him right in.

People made him nervous. He preferred dogs to people. That's how he supported himself and Buena. He raised hunting dogs and sold them to hunters. They would see his classified ad, make deals through the mail, and Buena would take the dog to town for him, collect his money. He didn't go to town with her because he slept all day. At dusk he would leave the house, run the dogs, and track animals until morning. Every night he took a paper sack of fried chicken with him, and around midnight, while the dogs howled, he would eat his one meal of the day.

He thought the doctor noticed that he smelled like his dogs, but she smiled when she greeted him and didn't seem to mind. She quickly got serious. She told him he was having a heart attack.

He didn't remember his first 2 days in the hospital. The doctor later told him that his heart had stopped, that he had actually died. When he woke up two days later, the aching in his arm was gone, but beneath his left collarbone he noticed a tube that looked like a yellow octopus with its head buried. His chest no longer felt like it was caving in on him, but whenever he took a deep breath, a knife hit him under the ribs. He felt weak. Something sucked out his energy like a tick sucks out blood. His skin smelled like soap. He realized they had cut his toenails.

He couldn't eat their baked fish and broccoli. He didn't eat for 2 days, until one of the night nurses talked to Buena and disregarded the doctor's orders out of pity. Buena brought him a brown paper bag filled with cold fried chicken, and he huddled over it like a hound dog and ate behind the drawn curtain. From then on they called him "the chicken man."

The next day he decided to leave. The doctor told him he might die, but his mind was set, and Buena brought him his clothes. The doctor gave him medicines, told him to take them, told him they were important. He left in a wheelchair, his feet aching in boots that no longer fit.

They stopped at a drugstore on the way home, but Buena came out and told him the medicines cost $60, that she would have to go home first and get more money. He told her to forget the pills, that he felt better without all those pills. As they drove further up into the clear mountain air, he assured her he was feeling much better. That night he was too tired to go out with his dogs, but when he tried to lay down he felt like he was smothering, as though he were breathing oxygen through a plastic mask. He fell asleep in the chair and dreamt that the dogs mistook him for a raccoon. He tried to run in his dream, but weariness overcame him, so he sat down against a tree and waited for the hunter's bullet to pierce his tired heart.

Life Care at Golden Acres

M. Andrew Greganti, MD

Life care communities for the elderly have increased in popularity, largely because of the sense of security they offer. But there is another side. What follows is from one of my wisest teachers, an elderly life care community resident. Her story:

*I*t seemed the right decision for Jim and me. We were most concerned about maintaining our independence as long as possible, but we needed to know that someone would be there when we could no longer care for ourselves. Both of us wanted not to burden our children with our problems. As a life care community, Golden Acres promised everything we could possibly need—a beautiful, rustic setting, on-site health care at all levels—nurse practitioner home visits, a convenient outpatient clinic, sheltered living, skilled nursing care in a well-run health center, and, most of all, the chance to meet new friends who, like us, were trying to cope with the challenges of growing old.

It would be expensive, but Jim and I had worked hard for our financial security. We had the money. Why not use it? It's hard to believe now, but 8 years have passed since we sold our home of 50 years and moved to Golden Acres.

The transition was more difficult than we had expected. Leaving long-term friends for a strange new place is never easy, especially with most of life behind you. But Jim and I somehow got each other through the rough spots. This time we were helped by a whole new set of friends, Golden Acres residents who knew too well what we were going through.

Our lives gradually began to return to normal. In many ways we began to enjoy ourselves. There were social events—plays to attend, invited speakers and informal social gatherings. And our new friends were interesting, from a variety of backgrounds—former academics, business executives, journalists. Clearly, our new circle did not represent a broad socioeconomic spectrum. However, it did represent a group of loving, caring people who could afford to live in this small microcosm of geriatric society. We would make the most of the time we had left and were convinced that this was the best place to do it.

Jim and I were not prepared for Linda's death. One rarely is. We ate with Sam and Linda almost nightly. Sam did most of the talking. In truth, Linda seemed hesitant to speak unless specifically asked for her opinion. She often appeared anxious in social settings and sometimes complained that she couldn't remember the names of her closest friends. Jim and I had also noticed that she frequently repeated herself. How could we have known she would shoot herself?

Linda's death made me notice the many widows and widowers at Golden Acres. Would Jim or I go first? What would I do without him or he, without me? Sam was facing these questions much sooner than he thought he would. Initially, he did as well as one could expect. Slowly, he began to withdraw, rarely eating in the dining hall and seldom coming to social gatherings. He lost weight, 30 pounds during the 6 months after Linda's death. Although his doctors diagnosed depression as the likely cause, further medical evaluation confirmed one of our worst fears—cancer.

"Why so soon after losing Linda?" Jim often asked, as if I would have the answer.

Over the next 4 years Linda and Sam's story would repeat itself more times than I would care to remember. It seemed that Jim and I would hardly get to know some of our new friends before we had to cope with their loss. Someone recently likened living in a life care community to sitting in "God's waiting room."

It's probably unfair to be so negative, to make it seem that all of us were totally preoccupied with death and dying. After all, Jim and I had found so many advantages. Perhaps the most notable was the reassurance that comes when you know you will be treated with respect and dignity no matter what your misfortune. We would never be alone; our many friends and the staff would see to that.

We continued to have many fun times together. Most of us had the means to live life to the fullest, and most did. For the first time in our lives, Jim and I could travel to places we had only dreamed of before. We took full advantage of the on-site physical fitness facilities, including an exercise room and swimming pool. But most of all we simply relished the opportunity to be among such an intellectually stimulating group of people.

In fact, so many things were going so well that Jim's stroke 3 years ago caught me off guard, at least psychologically. Subconsciously, I had begun to think that we had beaten the odds. Seeing Jim unconscious in the emergency room brought me back to reality. I knew that things would never be the same. Jim was left speechless with his right side totally paralyzed. Worse still, he was unable to comprehend verbal instructions and other conversation. He seemed to shun visitors, including me.

My trips to the Health Center became more difficult. It was bad enough to see my husband totally helpless. Worse still, I had to cope with seeing so many other people my own age devastated by one horrible problem or another. I had seen all of it before while visiting friends, but somehow I had to face it head on now that Jim had become a permanent Health Center resident. There was Sara next door walking aimlessly from one room to the next, often coming in and taking clothes from Jim's closet as if they were her own. I also got to know Tom who was regularly retrieved by the nurses after he triggered the alarm system trying to escape from what he could no longer understand. My thoughts were often preoccupied with the idea that some fates are truly worse than death.

I had plenty of support. The kids called and visited regularly, and our friends couldn't do enough. Nevertheless, I remained very uneasy. How much time should I spend with Jim? Did he really know the difference? Would the nurses take good care of him when I wasn't there? How long could this last? Then I had to cope with the guilt engendered by my wishing that Jim would die, for his sake and mine.

Jim had asked the same questions long before when we had visited friends at the Health Center. He had always feared lingering in a helpless state. Thank God, he didn't. Four months later he died of pneumonia. The children and I were thankful that his suffering had ended.

All in all, I guess I have been very fortunate. My health at age 85 remains good, and I am still able to remain very active by most standards and to enjoy my family and friends. But I would be less than honest if I didn't acknowledge more than a little ambivalence about the decision Jim and I made to move to Golden Acres.

Is it wise to compress so many of the problems of aging into such a small social unit? In many ways it is like watching the same movie 100 times. For many of us the known can become more feared than the unknown. Linda had seen several of her friends go through all the stages of Alzheimer disease. She knew she did not want to live through even the first stage and saw suicide as the only way out. Like Linda, will other residents of life care communities increasingly choose this alternative? I suspect so. The other day I was not surprised to hear one of my best friends wish for a hypothetical euthanasia chamber to allow those who wanted to end their lives to do so "with dignity." At first I thought she was joking. She was very serious indeed.

If given a second chance, would I decide to live at Golden Acres? I don't know. Life care communities offer more advantages than disadvantages, particularly when one becomes dependent on others for daily care. Certainly Jim and I were initially attracted to the availability of so many support services within a small geographic area. Convenience and easy access seemed so important at the time. Only later did we come to know the down side, the daily exposure to friends forced to endure all of the worst aspects of dependence. For both of us, the Health Center became the symbol of a fate we hoped to avoid at all costs.

A Job Well Done?
J. Randall Curtis, MD

Sitting here in the intensive care unit, waiting quietly while friends and family gather around the bedside to say their final good-byes to Paul, I find myself staring blankly out the window. The mechanical whir of the ventilator and the cold December rain on the window help me to drift peacefully back over the last two and a half years.

Paul was 23 years old when he and I first met. It was a warm July day in Seattle. I was in the first month of my internship, and it was Paul's first visit to my clinic. He had been healthy all his life, until the previous month when he landed in the hospital with bacterial pneumonia. He did well, spending only 36 hours in the hospital, and was referred to my clinic for follow-up care. As I rounded the corner to the examination room, the first I saw of him was his black, pointed-toe, suede boots propped up on my desk. When I introduced myself, standing formally with right hand outstretched, he slipped his feet slowly off the desk, put his Rolling Stone magazine in his canvas shoulder bag, and offered his hand, but didn't stand. I felt the contrast between his floppy blond curls hanging down around his round gold-rimmed wire glasses and my close-cut carefully combed brown hair; his oversized gray sweatshirt and my shirt and tie. Yet I remember feeling put at ease by his warm smile and attentive blue eyes. Because his medical history was short, we had plenty of time to cover nonmedical issues. He worked as a chef at a local restaurant but wanted to open a restaurant of his own in a few years. His restaurant was going to be such a success that he would be able to open a new one every time he felt ready to move to a new city. His last restaurant was going to be on one of the San Juan Islands where he and his lover would retire.

He seemed very comfortable telling me he was gay but added quickly that he had practiced safe sex since 1982 and had been in a monogamous relationship for the last 5 years. He had never had an HIV test, mostly because he didn't think he was at high risk. I talked him into having HIV serologic testing. Much can be done these days—even before any symptoms appear, I remember saying. I expected the result to be negative but wanted to be reassured because of his recent pneumonia.

He returned a week later. I greeted him cheerfully in the hall and went off to find his chart while a nurse put him in an examination room. When I found his chart and his HIV results, I had to sit down alone for a few minutes to collect my thoughts. I hadn't received any training on how to tell a 23-year-old that his dreams and hopes may have to take on an entirely new time frame: that he would probably never own a restaurant or retire in the islands. I remember hoping that he wouldn't break down and cry in my office—more for my sake than his. I also remember wanting to let him place his hope in the possibility that the test was wrong, but that didn't seem fair. Somehow we both got through that next half hour.

Over the next 2 years, Paul and I saw a lot of each other. There were spells when we saw each other once a week. Often he would come to clinic just to express his fears and anxieties; his friends and family sometimes found it difficult to listen to his anguish. Most of all, he feared the loss of freedom that he'd seen bedridden friends experience. At first, I would try to hide my discomfort when he talked about being afraid or when he cried. With time, I learned to listen without withdrawing or trying to talk him out of his pain. Eventually, I gave him my home phone number and he would sometimes call me there with urgent questions or simple worries.

He called me at home about a year ago; a close friend had died several days earlier and Paul had just returned from the memorial service. Paul called, he said, to ask me about some sores in his mouth. The pauses in his conversation made me suspect that the mouth sores were not his main concern. When I asked about his friend, he told me the story of a carefree young artist with progressive dementia, many of whose friends had pulled away in the last weeks. Paul resented those friends, his friends, who had stopped going to the hospital. Yet each time Paul went to the hospital to meet the unrecognizing eyes and to hear the incoherent ramblings, his anguish and sense of futility grew. He would dread each visit and then would chastise himself for his feelings. At first I tried to ease his guilt, but when my words met with a cool reception, I realized that wasn't what he wanted. Instead, I listened. The next time I saw him the crisis had passed and the mouth sores had healed. Paul thanked me more for the mouth rinse than for the time we had spent talking, but it wasn't the mouth rinse prescription that made me feel most like Paul's doctor.

Paul called me at home 3 weeks ago to tell me that his usual low-grade fevers were now up to 102° and that he was having trouble catching his breath. I admitted him that night, and he hasn't been home since. Once in the hospital, he seemed to get worse quickly. It wasn't long before Paul and I had to talk about intubation. Even then, Paul had a sharp mind and a knack for asking questions for which there were no answers. I talked in percentages and survival rates; Paul talked in time left to be with friends. Finally, we decided we would intubate him if we had to, but he made me promise that if the outlook became dismal, we would make him comfortable and turn off the machines. Two days after his decision, he was intubated.

There was a flurry of activity about Paul's bed for his first few days in the ICU: Consulting residents, fellows, and attendings came and went. Their experience and their technology were called into action, but, in Paul's story, it was the disease that was most persistent. The consultants have since drifted away—in part because they had little left to offer.

The outlook is dismal. He has been intubated for almost 2 weeks. I can't talk with him anymore, but he writes some and still has those crystal clear blue eyes.

Sitting here in the ICU, staring out blankly at the drizzling gray sky, I realize that I feel content. I'm sad, although perhaps not as sad as I was that day when I saw Paul's HIV results and felt an iron door slam shut on his future. Sad, but also proud of my role in Paul's life. I couldn't save his life, but I worked hard to give him as much time as possible. Not time spent exhausted and unable to get out of bed, but time to be with friends, to enjoy a breeze, or to cook a meal. When his last infection came, I acted quickly and aggressively in hope of giving him more time. But now it is clear that this is not the type of time we were fighting for, and I am prepared to stop. Not to stop giving my support and comfort. Not to stop spending time with Paul. But to stop trying to prolong his life. To some, this would be a failure. To me, for better or worse, this was a job well done.

Walking the Dog

She weighed
three hundred pounds.
Fat and high sugars
were killing her,
I thought.

So,
I thought.
So.

I gave her a puppy
with dark curly hair;
nothing else
had worked.

Walking the dog
twice a day,
I thought
might persuade,
might motivate.

She was pleased
with my prescription,
she laughed,
she rocked
from side to side.

She lived
for twelve years
hugging
that little black dog
while her lean husband
walked it faithfully,
twice a day.

                John L. Wright, MD

Board Questions
Michael A. LaCombe, MD

I can't exactly tell you when it was she entered the room. It was, I think, sometime between Infectious Disease and Rheumatology. We were hard at it, pounding out another certifying examination, and I can tell you this: Nineteen of us sitting around the table were stopped in our tracks by her entry. Nineteen of us set aside the nuances of synthesis and judgment, of multiple choice and true-and-false, and stared. (There was a 20th, who was himself so tangled up in a particularly convoluted question that he remained oblivious to her.)

She walked in as if she owned the place. She seemed totally in control of herself, unfazed by our presence. Nor was the aura about her projected by any particularly commanding beauty, the way a woman of startling appearance can command a room merely by being in it. Her appearance being what it was, it was quite the opposite with her. What was it then?

She had her household, her entire world balanced on her shoulder, all the clothes she owned, stuffed into an oversized yellowed sweatshirt bulging at the nape. She had gathered and held its waist to form the most rudimentary of backpacks. Her hair was hacked and shorn. Her body held none of the lean fitness so fashionably displayed by the hotel guests mingling out in the courtyard. Rather, she seemed thin, brittle, ill. And there was something about her skin that wasn't just right. There was an affliction here you couldn't put your finger on. She wore a faded green flannel shirt that hung below her hips over worn blue slacks which, in turn, fell straight to the floor, shapeless, cuffs dragging, almost obscuring her sandals— all of which served only to magnify rather than to conceal her infirmity.

We were holding our meeting in the Garden Room bordering on an inner courtyard shaded by palm trees and skirted by some species of aster I couldn't identify. This woman (the management would later tell us) had apparently gained entry to the courtyard through the parking lot abutting the ocean. She had come in through the north walkway along the stand of eucalyptus. Neither the opulence nor dress nor manner nor notice of the moneyed guests in the courtyard could stop her. The Garden Room had been declared off-limits by signs shouting *Private Party* and *Quiet! Board Meeting in Progress*. It didn't matter. We had left the door open, partly to fill the room with fresh California air, partly to admit the sounds and smells of freshly mown grass in January, and partly to delude ourselves into thinking that we too were vacationing, rather than in reality hunched around a table hewing and shaping some antiseptic formal written examination.

It wasn't her boldness alone that struck me. Anyone hungry enough, anyone driven by the sort of want she must have been suffering from, could easily have run the gauntlet she did. What bothered me, or impressed me rather, was her poise. She didn't just grab a handful of the Danish and make a run for it as I might have done. Rather she strolled up and down the buffet some 20 feet distant from our meeting table, calmly examining the feast before her. A mound of fruit heaped up and slid over in a cascade of melon, mango, and papaya. She peered at it, leaning this way and that without touching anything and then casually moved on as would an overly particular European housewife at market—shrewd, critically selective. The confectionery pastries were next in line, arranged in geometric fashion on a huge platter, largely left behind by us (mostly out of guilt I might add). This choice too she rejected, picking instead the large yeast-baked muffins none of us had been able to resist. Gently she set her load on the floor, split a muffin with her thumbs and spread healthy slabs of softened cream cheese on each half. This operation she managed with extreme care, with a correctness. She might have been sculpting clay for the art show on 82nd Street or melding oil colors on a spattered palette. This was no slapdash application by one half-starved. When she had finished her preliminaries, she topped each half with a thinly sliced filet of pink salmon. She had it right. She was nutritionally correct.

She balanced the two open sandwiches in one palm, lifted her household onto a shoulder and strolled out, to stand just outside the Garden Room door, face full to the midmorning sun (which was more than any of us had been able to do). She did not bolt with her stolen goods. She seemed above stuffing the folds and pockets of her baggy clothing with rolls and pears and packets of marmalade. She took no more than she had needed for the moment, and then stood there, warming herself in the sun, at brunch.

I surveyed my colleagues. They were transfixed. None of them had made a move. They regarded her with a mixture of amusement, pity, and awe. I saw our endocrinologist examine the woman with her piercingly intelligent eyes and it seemed that I could almost see her thoughts. Why was this woman so wasted? Was this diabetes undiagnosed, poorly controlled? Panhypopituitarism—that might be it. Images of trophic hormones and releasing factors filled the air. Now it was the gastroenterologist's turn. What was so peculiar about her complexion? There was a disease about her, not the attractive soft coffee-brown of the islands but rather the off-gray color of . . . hemochromatosis perhaps? Yes, that was it: bronze diabetes and a cirrhosis-studded liver, joints swollen, arthritic—poor soul! To the rheumatologist this was ochronosis. Where were the blue sclera, the pigmented cartilage? The cardiologist saw only cyanosis. To him this was an Eisenmenger's pure and simple, a VSD too long not listened for, a shunt now reversed, the step-up gone, the situation hopeless.

The room became filled with feeling, with a richness not there before. There was that uncommon fulfillment one feels just after a particularly stirring concert or an extraordinary three-act play, where you, the audience, feel moved and changed. The woman remained oblivious to us. She finished with her brunch, lifted her load, and turned to go. She stumbled, tottered under her load. The cardiologist half rose in his chair. The geneticist gripped the arm of the oncologist. I looked around the room again. The interest in her went beyond the academic, and even among the stiffest of academicians rose the old stirrings of the clinician. No longer were these deans, editors, scientists of the highest order. Suddenly they were doctors again. They wanted to help. They needed only to be asked and they would give it, the old-fashioned doctor-way.

I couldn't help myself. I went to the window to watch her leave. She picked her way through the throngs of honeymooners, vacationers, and idle rich, walking toward the sun and the courtyard exit. Where did she get that poise, that simple dignity? Was she living in some thought-disordered world? Did she believe herself to be Queen of the Tropics? Or was she absolutely on the mark, knowing that she had been among physicians, was a patient, and so, eminently superior to us? Could this have been a simple lesson in humanity: that she had nothing at all to be ashamed of, nothing for which to be scorned, that she was an equal among us, and belonged?

Misunderstanding

Morning rounds, the intern's order.
Discontinue TLC,
a word and three letters puzzling to me,
displayed so near approaching death
and this cold robot of volume and flow
quantitating every breath.
How inappropriate, it seems,
to discontinue tender loving care
for this spare woman scored with tears—
strange enough for me,
embarrassed to inquire of love
with a stethoscope tickling my ears,
to ask her nurse
the meaning of this doctor's order.

Oh, she reported,
that's Triple Lumen Catheter in this ICU.

So, now I understand
the meaning of TLC in room 262,
where we are headed this morning,
what a difference three letters can make
how much
the language of this work has changed.

                    Eric L. Dyer, MD

Ode to Joy
Mark S. Litwin, MD

When you've gone through the 4-year fire of medical school and you've walked the wards as a surgical intern, you think you're ready for anything. You think you can do anything. You learn to cut silk on the first try, tie knots with sutures fine as hair and list the causes of hypokalemic alkalosis. You can drive an IV into a veinless arm, hold a retractor, arms numb, for hours without moving. You can find any x-ray and summarize a 2-month hospitalization in less than 5 minutes. You become case-hardened, tough.

One patient can prove you wrong. Mrs. Bingham, on her 83rd birthday, arrived for surgery for a chronically infected toe. Despite her stroke and her limited vocabulary, she wore a perennial grin. Her Alzheimer disease had frayed her edges, but still she cooperated with the preoperative rituals we had in store for her. And how could I quarrel with an aphasic patient who arrived with a freshly typed medical history, a medication list, and a signed surgical consent form all packaged in the envelope from the nursing home? Mrs. Bingham had just saved me an hour.

The next morning I assisted in removing Mrs. Bingham's badly infected toe in a brief operation we were certain would improve her overall medical condition. Later that evening when I stopped by to check on her, she was sleeping peacefully, seemingly grateful that the surgery was over. As I stood watching her, her eyes slowly opened and a gentle smile broke across her face. Without words she seemed to tell me to tend sicker patients, that she was fine. I checked her dressing, stalled a minute to be with her, and then walked out of the room feeling uplifted, happy to be in medicine. I hurried off to other duties.

In the early morning dawn, the hospital takes on a certain quiet stillness. The lights are dimmed, the bustle has gone, and the pulse of the building slows down like that of a sleeping giant. But this seeming peace can be shattered in seconds. At 3:00 a.m. a nurse found Mrs. Bingham unresponsive in bed. The alarms screeched through the halls. The code sounded. All calm was transformed into a riot of respiratory therapists, EKG technicians, IV teams, messengers, nurses, interns and residents. We struggled with her for an hour, but in the end lost the battle. I was given the duty to phone her attending surgeon. He asked me to call the family.

Stop-the-code. The words echoed endlessly in my mind as I dialed Mrs. Bingham's son. In that instant, I felt the whole thing impossible. I had to tell her son, but I just couldn't do it on the phone. I lied. I asked him to come straight-away to the hospital, told him that his mother's condition had worsened. I then left the ward and paced the halls, finding myself not wholly accidentally at the intensive care unit where I might talk to Joy, the night shift supervisor. She could tell us interns what a patient needed without talking down to us. She had been a nurse long enough to know how to guide us gently through the most difficult nights of sick patients and on early morning rounds when the senior resident praised the interns' informed nocturnal decisions, Joy smiled to herself and winked from across the room as she left for the day. We had all learned this: Joy was the interns' friend.

"You look sad my friend," said Joy as I walked into the unit. She took me into her office and I told her the situation. *What would I say to this son*, she asked me. I shook my head. She sat me down and told me of some of her own experiences with families at times like this. She told me that although they might not ask, the children would want to know that their mother did not die in pain. She helped me sort my emotions so that I could show my feelings without being driven by them, and as I sat absent of the doctor's aura, human, she held my hand and helped me find strength. Joy prepared me for the most painful job I had yet to endure.

When the floor nurse paged to announce that the Bingham family had arrived, Joy asked me if I wanted her to go along. I nodded and we headed for the elevator. My heart pounded. I was filled with apprehension, covered with sweat. There they sat in the patient lounge on the 15th floor. At this time of such sudden intense intimacy what could I say to them? How could I confront them with the awful news. I had only my own experience to guide me. With Joy at my side, I told them that while Mrs. Bingham had come through the operation successfully, her weak heart had finally yielded to a greater power. I explained that she had quietly closed her eyes and drifted peacefully into a sleep from which she would never awaken.

But her son seemed relieved, as though I had lifted a burden and not created one. I took his hand and held it as tightly as Joy had held mine. The three of us, Joy, the son and myself, walked together to Mrs. Bingham's room. Her son kissed his mother's hand and knelt at the bedside to say good-bye. Then he thanked me, and calmly left. My teeth bit into my tongue as I fought back the tears and tried to retain my composure. On the elevator, utterly exhausted, I collapsed into Joy's arms and wept. She held me tightly, and told me what a fine doctor I was, how great my compassion. And at that November moment of my internship, I became a physician.

Your Name Escapes Me

Like polished pebbles worn smooth,
aging neurons no longer sift
and store memories but flow them past
unhindered as through a sluice
leaving murky puddles as residue.

Conrad Rosenberg, MD

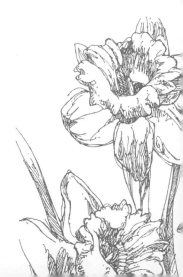

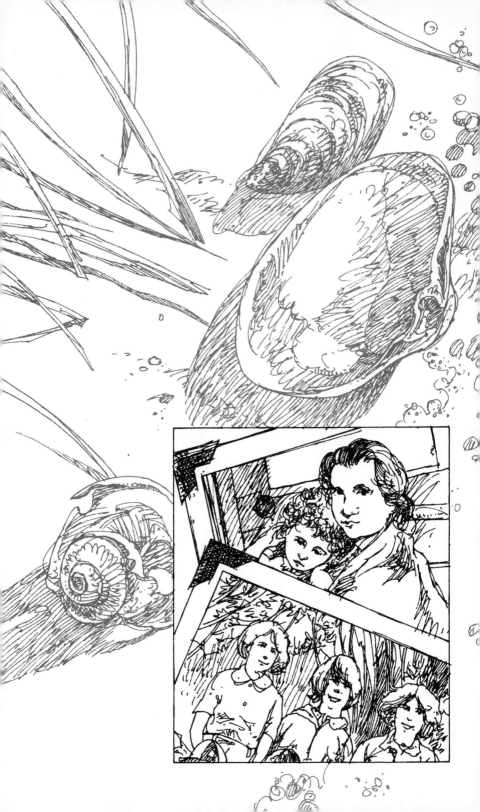

He Confronts Death

"My Grandmother's Illness" *from* The Guermantes Way

We may, indeed, say that the hour of death is uncertain, but when we say so we represent that hour to ourselves as situated in a vague and remote expanse of time, it never occurs to us that it can have any connexion with the day that has already dawned, or may signify that death—or its first assault and partial possession of us, after which it will never leave hold of us again—may occur this very afternoon, so far from uncertain, this afternoon every hour of which has already been allotted to some occupation . . . you have no suspicion that death, which has been making its way towards you along another plane, shrouded in an impenetrable darkness, has chosen precisely this day of all days to make its appearance.

Marcel Proust

A Birth in Tedda
Richard M. Hodes, MD

$\mathcal{G}$ had been in Tedda, a village in the northwest highlands of Ethiopia, for months, caring for several thousand Ethiopian Jews passing through a transit camp en route to Israel. They walked through mountain highlands and malarial lowlands for up to 3 weeks, armed and traveling in groups for protection from bandits and wild animals. The camp was a grassy site of a few acres, with residents living in tents, shelters, and papyrus huts. There were few amenities except for a small clinic. It was a two-bedroom cottage with a cement floor, cold water, and a Western toilet, making it the most modern building in the village.

Friday was quiet. In the evening I lit Sabbath candles with the children and invited the residents into the clinic for Kiddush, blessing the Sabbath wine. There had been no electricity for several days, and most people retired early. Saturday was blazing hot, and we slept all afternoon.

The early evening calm was broken when someone came in to inform me of a sick woman. I asked him to bring her to the clinic. Most of the people had no experience seeking medical care and had never seen a physician. We constantly encouraged them to come in when they were ill. My job was to treat their malaria, tuberculosis, scabies, and malnutrition and to keep them well. Childbirth was a particular challenge. In their villages, births were assisted by local women, trained or otherwise. I was not confident in their skills and knew that sterile technique was nonexistent. At the same time, as an internist with a bit of obstetric training, I felt that my own skills were limited to normal deliveries.

When the patient hadn't arrived in a few minutes, I wandered around the camp until I located her. Zewdie was a 20-year-old woman, pregnant with her second child, lying on the dirt floor of her canvas tent, surrounded by four or five relatives. They lifted her and guided her along a path to the clinic.

A dozen people followed her in; most were relatives but others were curious and simply wanted to observe. I promptly ordered everyone out so I could examine the patient and deliver the baby. Zewdie and three women remained: Birtukan Fassika, the 60-year-old daughter of Kes Fassika, a well-known rabbi from the Semien Mountains, and two others. All were dressed in traditional clothes: loose hand-woven white cotton dresses with colorful, embroidered designs along the borders. Birtukan's worn brown skin was well-lined, bespeaking her years. She had short gray hair covered with a black cloth which smelled of the pungent eucalyptus smoke of her cooking fires. Birtukan's one upper tooth fit perfectly into a gap in her well-stocked lower jaw. Around her neck she wore two metal beads on black threads as well as two strings of thin white beads.

Alemu, my health assistant, had walked into the village to eat, leaving me alone. Zewdie alternately squatted on her bed or lay on the right side. In Amharic, I asked her to lie on her back. She ignored me. I gently eased her onto her back and examined her. She was about 6 centimeters dilated, not yet ready to deliver. I felt frustrated by the paucity of support, Zewdie's lack of cooperation, and my own limited obstetric skills.

The electricity returned and I put on some water to boil ("just like in the movies," I thought), planning to tie the cord with dental floss and cut it with a boiled razor blade. The women had far different plans that excluded me. The brief exam I had undertaken without explanation did nothing to improve our relationship. Attempting to regain control, I asked Zewdie to lie on her back and eventually shouted and pounded the mattress, all to no avail. A crowd had gathered outside listening to us.

Alemu returned and produced an infant suction, thread, and a sterile blade, then cut the corner of a clean blanket in which to wrap the baby. Birtukan realized what we were doing and calmly handed me a razor blade and a piece of twine. Neither was very clean, but nonetheless she was prepared. The patient was kneeling, leaning forward with her arms around the neck of another woman, Birtukan sat on the bed behind the patient with her hand supporting Zewdie's buttocks. Alemu explained to the women that we wanted the patient on her back so we could assist the birth.

Birtukan, clearly the designated birth assistant, looked up. "This is not for men," she said firmly.

I was not permitted to touch the patient. Zewdie moaned during her periodic contractions as I stood by. I felt helpless and impotent, controlled by an illiterate, homespun midwife. My anger was increasing and I considered forcing Birtukan and the others out so I could take charge. Zewdie's choice, however, was obvious. I reluctantly backed off.

A short time later, the contractions slowed. Birtukan announced that she needed a "kai doro" and "itan." I wondered if I heard her correctly asking for a doro (chicken). I was astounded when one of her assistants soon entered carrying a live, red, squawking chicken upside-down by its legs. As Zewdie leaned forward, Birtukan took the chicken in her right hand and made large circles with the bird's breast against Zewdie's back. Another messenger entered and showed me a yellow, crystalline substance wrapped in an old newspaper.

"Itan," Alemu commented quietly, "frankincense."

Smoking coals on a metal grate were brought in, and the frankincense was added. The room immediately filled with thick, pungent smoke. Birtukan continued making silent circuits with the bird in a businesslike manner. I quickly opened the window to prevent us from being asphyxiated. As the air cleared, Birtukan turned to me. "This will speed the labor," she said, as a teacher speaks to a new student.

Before she finished her explanation, the baby crowned. Zewdie was kneeling steadily on her hands and knees. I immediately gloved and caught the baby boy, moving him away from a pool of amniotic fluid on the plastic mattress. He breathed easily and his color was good. As Alemu and I clamped the cord, Birtukan and her assistants put a shawl over Zewdie's back to block the baby from the crowd of people watching at the doorway. Alemu appeared nervous as he tied and cut the cord, and his usually steady hands trembled. He had done this many times, however, and I did not comment.

We laid the baby on a piece of cut blanket and waited for the placenta. I was relieved that things had gone smoothly thus far. I always feared an abnormal presentation. This time it would have been more difficult because of Birtukan's presence and my marginal role in the birth. Birtukan called for "gunfo," a thick mixture of oil and boiled wheat for the mother to eat.

With the stress of the delivery behind me, I wanted to understand Birtukan's techniques.

"Birtukan, why the chicken?" I asked.

"Koleh, an evil spirit," she explained, "separates the patient from God and slows the birth. We use the red chicken and incense in every birth to block the Koleh."

"But," I asked, "what happens if the baby still doesn't come?"

She looked up. "Then you have to stand the pregnant woman up." She stood to imitate the position. "You keep her standing, but make her bend as far forward as possible from the waist, grabbing her ankles with her arms and keeping her head down by her knees. Then two men must pick her up by the legs and shake her. If that doesn't work," she continued, "you have to turn the woman upside-down and shake her some more. Then you point her head toward the floor and gently shake her again. Keep it gentle. After doing this several times, instruct her to squat. This will rotate the baby if it is in an abnormal position."

Birtukan admitted that although she had delivered countless babies, she had used the more extreme maneuvers infrequently. I asked her how she got all her knowledge, and she replied that as a young girl she observed the older women in the village.

She looked over at Zewdie and added, "If this fails, I call in a more senior person."

"Who would be more senior than Birtukan?" I wondered.

"A few women," she went on, "put butter on their hands and insert them in the uterus to rotate the baby until it is in a position to emerge on its own."

Alemu called that the placenta had just been delivered.

"It looks good," I commented. Birtukan was behind me.

"Hulu wutual," she assured us, "It's all out."

As I bathed the baby, I asked Birtukan why she had held up a shawl while we cut the cord.

"Buda—evil eye," she replied. "A lot of people were watching. If any had evil eye, the baby would become sick." Ethiopian mothers often stay inside for weeks to protect their newborns from such things.

Word spread throughout the camp that the baby was born, a healthy boy. The room filled with women who brought fresh coffee made over fires lit after the Sabbath ended at nightfall. They painted Zewdie's hair with butter 12 times, each accompanied by high-pitched ululations.

The chicken squawking in Zewdie's room next to mine woke me before sunrise. I rolled over and asked myself, "Was it really necessary for a chicken to sleep in the clinic last night?" I walked into Zewdie's room to check the baby.

"Dam nebur," Birtukan announced without emotion, "there was some bleeding."

I saw that the baby was very pale and his blanket was soaked with blood. Birtukan had retied the cord with her twine. The baby was less active than he should have been. His skin showed signs of dehydration and his heart rate was slower than expected. It made no sense to me since I expected an increased heart rate from blood loss. I was confused and becoming nervous.

I woke the staff and we made an oral rehydration solution with extra sugar. The baby was now asleep, so I inserted a nasogastric tube, confirmed its position, and slowly gave fluid through a syringe. Soon after, he stopped breathing. Alemu carried him into the examination room and I began gentle chest massage and mouth-to-mouth breathing while he suctioned frothy fluid from the nose several times a minute.

The baby seemed cool. Alemu suggested we move into my bedroom which gets the morning sun. He picked up the baby and rushed him in, lying him on a clipboard on my bed to support compressions. I placed the baby in warm water and continued the process for several minutes, soaking myself and the floor. I couldn't believe this was happening. Last night this was a healthy newborn and an uncomplicated delivery. As I looked at him in the bath, something inside me said, "In a minute he'll wake up and be normal." When we transferred him to the bed, the frothy sputum coming from the lungs became blood-tinged, strongly suggesting pulmonary edema. I surmised that he had a congenital heart lesion. We continued resuscitation, but there had been no signs of life for over a half hour.

"Any suggestions?" I asked the staff.

Nobody volunteered. We all felt crushed. I thanked everyone and halted our efforts, almost 12 hours after his birth. A nurse went in to tell the mother that her baby had died. Loud wailing arose from the room next door.

I called for our regular morning prayers to begin and asked a few men to prepare a grave in the Tedda Jewish Cemetery, a remnant of the time when hundreds of Jews lived permanently in the village. I asked Birtukan to explain the burial custom. As an old woman and the daughter of a rabbi, she would certainly know how to prepare a body. She instructed me to wash it, tie together the wrists, thumbs, and ankles with twine, and cover it with "abujedi," a yellowish cotton in which Ethiopians wrap corpses. I followed her instructions, placed the body in abujedi, and sewed it shut.

Alemu wrapped a sheet of wicker around the abujedi. I noted how well Alemu tied knots in the wicker, then realized that he had tied the umbilical cord. At that moment, he paused, looked up, and said, "I'm sorry." I said I understood. I did not blame him and I was not convinced that blood loss was responsible for the baby's death.

I asked a young Ethiopian rabbi nearby to officiate at the funeral. He explained that when a newborn dies, it is their custom to bury the body without ceremony and without a rabbi. We carried the body to the cemetery, across dried ploughed fields, and up a hill. When we arrived at the site, we found the earth was hard and dry. The prepared grave was too small, so Alemu and I took picks and enlarged it.

I counted the mourners. There were nine men and an equal number of women. We could not say Kaddish, the prayer for the dead, without 10 men. Our worlds were far apart. Kaddish was my tradition, not theirs. So was sterile technique and barring animals from the delivery room. Despite this distance, I looked at these people with admiration and wonder. Their faith, strength, and tenacity had kept them together for centuries. Only with openness and respect for their traditions could I be successful with them. This meant considering Birtukan a colleague rather than an adversary and tolerating the chickens, ululation, and my limited role.

I felt calm but drained. I took the body and placed it in the grave. Several of us put handfuls of dirt on the corpse, then took turns filling the grave with a shovel. Afterwards, we placed a large pile of stones over the site to mark the grave.

It seemed too soon to leave. We all sat down. Alemu gave a talk. Then I said, "Dear God, we thank you for the birth of this baby, and we pray that you protect its soul, now and forever." Alemu translated. We sat for a few minutes more in silence. We were on a hill overlooking brown, rolling farmland. The sides of the hills were dotted with mounds of grain. Cows grazed in the distance. The wind blew gently on us. It was peaceful, idyllic. A baby on a woman's back cried as the mother shook her shoulders to amuse her.

"Ishi," I said, "OK."

We stood up and slowly filed out. The men carried their dulas, walking sticks or shovels or picks.

"Qoy, qoy," I called. "Wait a moment. I want to thank you for coming. Many of you are not related to the family at all. I appreciate your being here."

"Chiger yellem," they replied, "no problem," as they walked away.

Later I stopped into Birtukan's tent. She was sitting on the ground, chatting with a relative. "I know you feel very bad," she said to me. "We all feel that way."

"Birtukan, you're right," I replied. "How long will it last?"

She looked into my eyes.

"A week. A week, and that's it," she said confidently.

"How can you be so certain?" I asked.

"The Bible says so," she answered.

Informed Consent
Kenneth B. Wasser, MD

*B*obby's eyes would sparkle when he talked about baseball. He knew all the top players' batting averages dating back to their rookie years. Like a lot of 12-year-old boys, Bobby loved baseball. But unlike most, he never had a chance to play little league or sandlot ball. Bobby had muscular dystrophy. His delayed motor development, waddling toe walk, and large calf muscles made the diagnosis painfully obvious when he was still a toddler. Physical therapy, bracing, and heel-cord-release surgeries were futile in preventing Bobby from being confined to a wheelchair by the time he was 8. Now, at 125 pounds, his pear-shaped body was nearly impossible for his mother Susan to handle. Caring for him was a full-time job and she had little help at home. Bobby's father, unable to cope emotionally with the illness, had left them when the child was only 6. Although Susan was attractive with short, brown hair and an engaging smile, she was never able to find a companion willing to share her devotion to Bobby. She proudly displayed her community college degree on the walls of her apartment, yet she knew that working outside the home and entrusting Bobby's total care to someone else was financially and emotionally impossible.

Bobby had been in the intensive care unit before, but this time was different. Susan could barely stand looking at what seemed like an endless stream of lines and catheters going in and out of her beloved son. She realized Bobby's muscular dystrophy had severely damaged his heart muscle causing, as one of his doctors explained, "a severe cardiomyopathy unresponsive to conventional antiarrhythmics." With increasing frequency, the cardiac monitors would sound their alarms, the intensive care team would perform CPR, and Bobby would be defibrillated into normal sinus rhythm. This scene was repeated as if it were part of a Broadway show rehearsal. Susan also knew Bobby's respiratory muscles were losing what little power they had left. Her practiced eye could see by the movement of the respirator that Bobby was breathing less and less on his own. Although she knew the hopelessness of the situation, she could not bring herself to put an end to what she considered the hi-tech medical torture of her child. In the beginning, whenever the alarms went off, the doctors would ask Susan to leave the room. After a while, the ICU team let her stay with Bobby. From time to time, Susan was asked by a member of the medical team to consent to a "do not resuscitate" order. She never could. "How can I sign my child's death warrant?" she would ask. "Please don't ask me to do this."

Fortunately, Dr. Harold Jones was also involved in Bobby's care. Dr. Jones was tall, had a crop of white hair on each side of his bald crown, and walked with military bearing. He inspired immediate confidence. Despite his formidable appearance, he had the uncanny ability to establish rapport instantly with patients. He had seen Bobby from time to time in the muscular dystrophy clinic and they had gotten along fabulously because both of them loved the Boston Red Sox and could not stand the New York Yankees. Whenever Dr. Jones would talk to patients, he would always be at eye level, never looking down at them in their beds. He did not allow objects such as a desk to come between him and a patient. He would either sit down on the bed with the patient or pull up a chair alongside. He usually held the patients' hand and gently touched them wherever they felt the slightest discomfort. He didn't spend an excessive amount of time with people, but they always seemed to feel he was there longer than he actually was. Perhaps his empathy stemmed from his first-hand knowledge of loving a handicapped child. His own son was severely mentally retarded.

Dr. Jones sat with Susan, held her hand, and listened to her story. He agonized with her about her inability to consent to a "do not resuscitate" order. He felt the need to come between the bureaucratic, legal aspects of Bobby's care and Susan's personal struggle. Then it happened again. Bobby's head rolled sideways and the alarms sounded their continuous BEEEEP. Dr. Jones looked into Susan's pleading eyes and appeared to see into her heart. He stood up, blocked the doorway and prevented the intensive care team from entering. For a moment it seemed as if there would be a confrontation. But Dr. Jones was obviously immovable. He clearly had Susan's "informed consent" even though no papers had been signed or court orders issued. His authority to act in Susan's behalf went unchallenged. Susan held Bobby and sang him his favorite baseball song. She and Dr. Jones exchanged glances for the last time and then she whispered, "Thank you."

Core Curriculum
Jeffrey A. Katt, MD

*W*e all have had one patient we never forget. For me that patient was Helen. I was in my 4th month of internship and, like many of my colleagues, had doubts concerning my career choice of internal medicine. It seemed my patients never improved and were bouncing in and out of the hospital on a monthly basis. Yes, there was the occasional young patient with pneumonia who made a complete recovery, but it seemed that the patients I was most familiar with, those with chronic lung disease or congestive heart failure or diabetes or cancer, would often show only modest improvement, an improvement that seemed to last for less time with each successive hospitalization. I was chronically tired and irritable, and I began to wonder what the reason for this futility might be. It was at this point that Helen came into my life.

It was my first day on the oncology service, a rotation I had been dreading for weeks. Helen was my first assigned patient. She had been fighting a long, arduous battle against breast cancer, with multiple recurrences and repeated courses of chemotherapy. She came to the emergency room with fever, hemolytic anemia, fluctuating neurologic signs, and severe thrombocytopenia. She had thrombotic thrombocytopenic purpura. Because my service wasn't very busy, I found myself spending a great deal of time with Helen. She had recently moved to our locale after the death of her husband and had no friends or relatives in the area, no one to visit her. Helen was an exceptionally intelligent, courageous human being and always maintained her sense of humor. She understood her disease and frequently asked direct, specific questions about her prognosis, questions I found difficult to answer. We discussed her "code status" often, usually at her request. She was determined to live her life as fully as possible for as long as possible, despite her deteriorating condition.

The weeks went by. Helen and I came to understand each other. If it was a quiet night on call, I would stop by her room to play cards. I asked about her past, learned about a previous brush with death after an automobile accident in which her son was killed, her long career as a college professor, and the sudden and tragic recent death of her husband. I began to respect Helen, to admire her, and, even more, to like her.

Helen's condition worsened. She became confused. I could not raise her platelet count. One day in the midst of this, Helen begged me not to let her die. I felt helpless, guilty, knowing there was absolutely nothing I could do. The next day she asked her nurse to have me stop by again. She had changed her mind. She had had enough; she did not want her life prolonged in any way, should she continue to grow worse. The next day I confirmed her decision and reassured her that it was the right decision considering her stage of the disease. It was the first time I had seen Helen cry.

Three nights later, on call, I was summoned to Helen's room. She was short of breath, diaphoretic, and coughing. Each cough produced dark clots. Her chest x-ray suggested massive pulmonary hemorrhage, and I knew that Helen's time had come. I sat at the bedside holding her hand. She looked remarkably calm and accepting. She turned slowly to her nightstand and removed an envelope from the drawer. "Read it later," she said as she smiled weakly, handing it to me. Over the next hour, still holding her hand, I watched as she drifted in and out of consciousness and eventually stopped breathing. I pronounced her dead. The entire scene seemed to me strangely surrealistic.

I returned to the on-call room and opened the envelope. Her letter thanked me for my care and, more important, for my friendship, for caring about her. She was especially grateful for the kindness, respect, and friendship she had felt from me. I realized that way of treating her was the only aspect of her care that had come with little effort and also the only aspect of her care never mentioned or encouraged on my daily teaching rounds. I saved the letter, carried it in my pockets for weeks. It was the first time I cried over the death of a patient.

I've never forgotten Helen. She has changed the way I view patients. From her I learned that curing a disease is not always the most important aspect of the doctor-patient relationship. Patients visit their doctors for many reasons, sometimes for emotional support or kindness, for empathy and for openness, far more therapeutic than medications. Few things are more edifying than a patient who, despite having a deteriorating medical condition, seems to enjoy coming to the office. Since Helen, I treat all my patients with trust and respect, or try to, and perhaps more importantly, I treat them as equal human beings. And on those days when practice is especially difficult, when there seems no reward, I read Helen's letter again and remember that it is possible, no matter what the outcome, to make a difference in the life of a patient.

When a Heart Stops
Deborah L. Kasman, MD

*I*t was the summer of 1987 and the beginning of my last year of residency. Having easier rotations, I felt rested and wanted to earn some money. Northwest Emergency Physicians offered me a 24-hour shift at Moses Lake emergency room. It was a chance to earn good money and to travel to eastern Washington, the arid part of the state I had not seen since driving across the country 2 years earlier to begin my residency. Loving explorations, I accepted their offer.

The night before the journey my mind swam in excited and apprehensive thoughts as the minutes sped by. What cases would I see? Was I fully trained for my work? What were the people like in rural Washington? Finally, I dozed off. Three a.m. arrived before I knew it.

The lights of the city were low, and thick clouds covered the silent black Seattle sky. A cool breeze brushed my bare skin as I started my car and headed for the highway. I rolled the window down to wake up, rolled it up to warm up, and down again to feel alive and alert in the cold night air. After driving through mountain passes in total darkness, the soft rolling acres of farmland were a pleasant surprise in the morning light. Sprinklers filled the sky with a fine mist as cows grazed and tractors plowed. The Columbia River snaked through the countryside and I-90 stretched on forever.

I arrived at the small rural hospital just before 7 a.m. The staff greeted me warmly and gave a quick tour of the ER. They showed me their fully equipped treatment room, where the supplies were stored, and how to fill out billing slips. The nurse asked if I was tired from the drive and said, "It's usually quiet in the morning. Why don't you rest?"

I headed upstairs to the doctors' room for a nap. I was drifting off to sleep when the telephone rang.

"Get down here STAT. We have a head injury." Click. I shoved on my shoes, popped in my contacts, and raced down the stairs to the treatment room.

The scene was terrifying. One nurse pounded out chest compressions on a ghostly white boy while the respiratory technician squeezed the oxygen bag. I looked over my shoulder hoping to see another doctor. The hall was empty. I wanted to run away. The glaring hospital room with its whirring ventilator and anxious staff working on the boy filled me with dread. My heart and head began to pound.

"Page the pediatrician and the surgeon!" I shouted.

I placed my hand on the boy's cold wrist. I couldn't find a pulse. I came to my senses and started running his code.

I had never resuscitated a child before. This blond-haired boy looked about 10 or 11. Frantic—desperate—to revive him, I placed the paddles on his chest. The monitor showed a flat line.

"Everyone back," I shouted and delivered the shock. His small body jerked. There still was no heart rhythm.

"Continue CPR," I commanded. I recharged.

"Everyone back," I said and delivered another shock. He jerked again. Still no life rhythm.

"Epinephrine," I yelled. I called for intubation. The respiratory technician looked at me as though I were crazy. As air was pressed into the boy's lungs, half of it bubbled out of a huge crack in his skull. What could be left of his brain? I had to do something! As I watched his chest move up and down with the breaths delivered, I decided to start an IV line. Unable to feel a femoral pulse, I placed a large-bore needle into his cold, pasty skin, searching for a vessel. My needle came back dry. Maybe a subclavian! The chest compressions stopped me. I looked at the boy's outstretched form, then at the nurses. Three faces stared back at me. The senior nurse shook her head.

"What's the use?" I thought. I knew in my heart his soul had already left.

"You can stop now. Thank you for your help," I said. Everyone sighed—except me. I felt a pain I had never known before. My chest felt empty, as if my own heart had stopped . . . . I thought about his family. I had to tell his parents that their son was dead. Too late, the pediatrician came running in. She took one look at the boy, looked away, and left. She did not speak to me. She was gone, leaving me alone in this sterile room filled with antiseptic solutions.

Finally, I asked for the story. There had been a car accident 20 miles away on I-90—that long stretch of road that seemed so romantic to me earlier this morning. The same morning a family of five left Spokane on a trip with their two daughters in the back seat (wearing their seat belts) and their son on a mattress in the back of the van. Mom was driving while Dad slept in the passenger seat. The mother dozed. The van veered off the road and rolled over, throwing the boy from the van. His father ran to him and held him until a motorist stopped and sped them to the nearest hospital. The ER staff moved the boy, who had breathed his final breath in his father's arms, into the treatment room and began CPR.

The child was dead on arrival, and resuscitation was a long-lost dream. Could another doctor have saved him? This was the first time in my experience that an unstable patient arrived without an ambulance, without EMTs calling out vital signs and IVs running, without any hope of success.

I finally left the treatment room. The father was waiting in the counseling room across the hall. I did not know how to share my grief or express the adequate sympathy for his loss. I went in. The boy's father was a thin, fairly young man, with dark brown hair just starting to gray. He looked up at me with pain in his eyes.

"I am Dr. Kasman. We did all that we could, but it was too late. I'm sorry." He already knew. I gently touched his arm and asked if he wanted to see a pastor. "No, but thanks," he replied as he stared at his hands. His wife and daughters would arrive soon.

"Let me know if you need anything," I said quietly and left.

The staff now had several patients in exam rooms. I was it, "the doctor in charge," and I had more patients to see. Work waited as sick patients peered out of their rooms. These problems were easily handled.

After I saw a few patients, the automatic doors opened and the boy's mother, heavy with fear and loss, walked in. She saw her husband and ran to him and asked if he was all right. They clung to one another and cried. They held each other without blame, sharing only their sorrow. I showed the wife and daughters to the counseling room and asked if anyone was hurt. The wife had a few facial lacerations. The girls were uninjured.

I saw more patients. When the mother was ready, she was placed in a room. She lay still on the examining table with tears welling up. She bit her lip and whispered, "I fell asleep." I wanted to comfort her, but not finding the words, I busied myself. I numbed her skin with lidocaine and asked her to tell me if she was not fully anesthetized. She winced as I placed the first stitches but said nothing. She seemed to want to feel the pain. I injected more lidocaine to ease her physical pain.

"It's not your fault. I'm not here to hurt you," I said. She bit her lip harder and wept quietly. She asked me to check her daughters. Both were scared and shocked but physically unharmed. They returned to the counseling room to wait for their grandparents.

More patients. Six hours had passed since this tragedy began. Still, I was numb. The nurses mentioned lunch but I had neither the time nor the desire. I saw more patients. Finally, the grandparents arrived. The grandmother was a short, white-haired woman wrapped tightly in a long gray coat. She looked at me with inquiring eyes. She could not bring herself to hug her daughter. (Or was it her daughter-in-law?) The tension rose. Someone had killed her grandson. Was it me or the mother? Fortunately, they brought their own pastor to comfort them.

I saw more patients. Shortly after 1:30 the automatic doors opened again and the family began to leave. The parents embraced their daughters as they walked into the bright afternoon light. The glass doors slowly closed as they left their son's body behind, taking only his spirit home.

As I write this now my eyes fill with tears . . . tears I could not release then. There were more patients to see. My ordeal might be over but the day, and the anguish, were not. In the 17 hours to come, I slept only 2 hours and saw 40 patients. A 20-year-old man walked in with his scalp lifted from his forehead after he had play-fully jumped into a river bed that was too shallow. I secured his neck and applied pressure to his bleeding wound. I directed a nurse to start an IV as I clamped bleeder after bleeder. Finally I had the staff call a surgeon. The patient bled more; I clamped more. The surgeon arrived just as the field was dry. But now my ER was full. In the evening, a Hispanic migrant worker arrived in labor. Her only English was, "It's my time." She was only 29 weeks along. I stopped her contractions and had her airlifted by helicopter to a high-risk neonatal center.

"Will it ever end?" I wondered. Another patient was placed in a room.

The pace slowed as the night dragged on. I sunk more stitches, tended more coughs, and treated more stomach flus. The police brought in a rowdy drunk. My body craved sleep. I no longer cared about the money earned. The dark hours passed and morning finally came. My shift was finally over.

Despite the bright sunshine, I had to struggle to stay awake on the drive back to Seattle. I thought of my own vulnerability as my eyes tried to close and stopped only one-half hour from Seattle to buy soda and candy to keep me awake until I safely returned home. When I arrived, I called my parents, explained I had just completed a 24-hour ER shift, and quickly said good-bye. As I lay on my bed and stared at the ceiling, I saw that beautiful young boy, cheated from Little League games, from being teased by his sisters, from fishing with his dad, and from his first-date jitters. I wanted to be held. I seemed to cry for hours. Warm tears ran down my face and neck as I wept. Finally, sleep won, trapping my sorrow for years.

Yes, I talked about the boy's death. I shared it with other residents and with faculty. In the even light of day, we discussed how the boy was already dead and how I had done all that was possible. We reviewed the steps to have taken if the boy had had a pulse: how to intubate him and how to protect his spine. We learned the procedure for defibrillating a child and how to start an interosseous IV when indicated. Everyone said I had managed the situation well. They gave me their best support.

But no one asked how I felt.

Absolution

Wisps of gray
fanned across her pillow
a corona around a rose
replaced by a skeleton's mask,
her form made soft
by a snow-white patina
that touched her hills
and graciously unbroken
glided across her ravaged valleys.
At her center in dark hollows
a pair of sapphires,
and I immobilized.

In wispy voice she spoke:
You bend so wearily my friend.
Come, sit by me.
Recall our first meeting
how we browsed
your armory
planning our strategy
designing our tactics.

Give me your hand.
Forget thoughts of regret,
we are allies on the rock of reality.
I hated you
for failing;
but I love you for trying.

For a breath of time
you were my god,
now forever my friend.
You'll remember me,
and smile
at our audacity;
the battle lost
before we fired a shot.

She lay silent,
her chest barely moving
then said:
I feel sad
for you.
Soon I'll leave
but a shard of me
will be added
to that mountain of fragments
you awake to each day
knowing more will come.
I understand why you bend,
and I forgive
that you will live
and I will not.

The cold kiss
is upon my cheek.
It's time.
Hold me
then turn off the light,
I have no fear of the dark.

George Girey, MD

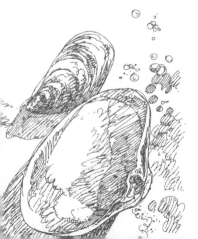

At the Sea's Edge

Come, dear pilot,
I would make my way to the salt sea,
For I have cried my fill,
And to all I ever loved
Have said goodbye;

What I could ever say
I have said,
What comfort I could take
From other hands
I have taken,

Unmoor me, now
And set me free,
I would range
Upon the roaming sea

Alone with dolphins and whales
To keep my company,
And all the rocking stars,
My light to be;

I hear the sea winds
Sing to me,
Like wind in the singing leaves
Of my beloved poplar tree,

That once sang me asleep.

Give me your hand
And my art shall comfort you,
Away from tired land
I shall carry you,

Roam, dear friend,
My heart shall cry for you,
And at day's end
I shall search for you.

And now I cry
Tears saltier than the sea;
Whose hands can comfort me?

Fred Coe, MD

Do Not Resuscitate

She held her mother's hand
and listened to the radio
Play "Country Roads." Their
Faded photo on the nightstand
Was still pleasant to look at.

Red, yellow, black. The
Bedsores came in various colors,
Shapes, sizes. Decaying flesh. And
The severed legs. Their remnants
Quivered when she was turned.

The feeding tube mocked death,
Leading into her stomach white
Liquid, and she mixed it
With a bit of gruel.
(She would only eat for her.)

She used to ask about
The grandchildren. Now even
The glimmer in her eyes
Was gone. And locked in her
Bed, so was the struggle.

"Prolong living, not dying,"
She knew full well;
But she longed for
A sign: Where was the
Dividing line?

"Every drop of life is
Precious," her father
Had said. "Savor every
Moment of it." And she
Remembered his smile.

She kissed her mother,
Released her hand,
Smoothed the fine hair,
And thought, wistfully,
"The end of life is also life."

Elliott Perlin, MD

What Have I Done?
Thomas M. Gill, MD

There's a code on 2 North!" a nurse with a high-pitched voice shouts from across the room.

I remove my stethoscope from the barrel chest of a middle-aged smoker. He had arrived at the emergency room of the local VA Hospital a few minutes before, in the early hours of a rainy, Pacific Northwest morning. Rubbing the vestiges of sleep from my eyes, I follow the nurse who had located me. Earlier in my training I may have raced to the scene, my pulse pounding and my mind muddled. But now I'm a grizzled warrior, not unlike these previously gallant veterans of war who have entrusted their medical care to me on this day. I proceed up the stairs and down the hall, carried by my weary legs into the room presently in turmoil.

The limp body of an elderly gentleman lies supine on a hospital bed, his skin dangerously ashen. No pulse; no respirations. The show begins: chest compressions to transport the stagnant blood; warm, moist oxygen to fuel the stricken corpus; one spark after another to awaken the quivering heart.

Who was this poor man anyway? Was he a Purple Heart recipient? Did he lead a charge up the hill at Iwo Jima? Maybe he served in Patton's Third Army as a combat infantryman. Is he now a proud grandfather or even great grandfather, the patriarch of a large prosperous family? Or is he an embittered recluse, sharing life with a jug of whiskey and a deck of cards? A quick review of his chart reveals only that he had been admitted the day before with a rapid heart rate and had been stabilized and transferred to a general medical ward to await further diagnostic evaluation.

Potent medications follow; fragments of an organized rhythm; an occasional spontaneous pulse to prod us onward. But the minutes roll on, relentless as the rain.

Now the body shakes vigorously in convulsion as if any remaining life is making a harried escape from all this madness. The eyes, previously a mint green, but now a dirty grey, have retreated deeply into the balding skull and have dilated and turned upward as if indicating their disapproval.

Another round of sparks and juice, but to no avail. Twenty minutes have passed. Dejected visages from the gallery await the next order even though they sense the battle has been lost.

"Any disagreement?" No. And efforts cease. The show has ended.

The time of death is . . . But wait . . . Yes! There's a pulse, bounding, seemingly in malicious contempt. On the monitor, a rhythm now compatible with life appears, but there are no spontaneous respirations. An endotracheal tube passes from my unsteady hand into the silent airway of the resurrected body and we speed away to the intensive care unit.

What have I done? On the surface, it appears that I have saved a life. But at what price? Too early to tell. Previous experience leaves me with serious doubts and misgivings. I am reminded of a study showing that less than 1 out of 10 patients over the age of 69 who had experienced a cardiopulmonary arrest while in the hospital survived to discharge. If the resuscitation had lasted more than 15 minutes, less than 1 out of every 100 survived; and of the survivors, most experienced serious functional and mental impairments, ranging from a partial paralysis to dementia or psychosis.

Should I have stopped my efforts sooner? Should they have begun in the first place? Unfortunately, but not surprisingly, the patient's wishes were not known; nor had they been requested. Would this poor man have consented to my assault on his person if he had been aware of the consequences? And does his soul, caught in a tangled web of technology, curse me now as I methodically write the very orders that may ensure its continued immurement?

The first sign of the reawakening is merely a withdrawal of a limb to a painful stimulus. It is enough, however, to revitalize my efforts and renew my hope. In confirmation of the rebirth, the eyes open slowly and the head nods hesitantly in recognition of its name.

Exhilaration, as I have never experienced before, and a sense of a new father's boastful pride well up within me as I look upon this miracle of medical science. "The exception that proves the rule," I tell my wife later that evening. I'm still wound tight as a spring when my head hits the pillow for the first time in nearly 40 hours.

Two weeks later, I'm back for another moonlighting shift. The sound of stomping feet passes my call room door. "All men to 2 North. A patient is out of control!" Turmoil once again. Arms flailing, voices shouting, a defiant glare from those same mint green eyes.

I linger at the door, the situation now well in hand. A raving lunatic is chained to a hospital bed by thick, rust-colored leather restraints coiled about each appendage. "He's never been the same," the head nurse explains as she scurries past me. Humbled and disheartened, I glance upward to acknowledge what I have done.

The Cause of Death

He died,
   and I do not know
   (nor ever will)
the cause of death.
A frail heart,
   too soon grown tired?
Just yesterday he smiled;
   a smile abruptly gone . . .

His care was in my hands;
And so I bear the consequences,
   the gnawing doubt
   forever unresolved:
   did I allow
   or (worse)
   bring on
   this death?
   Or was it serendipity,
   mere chance occasion?
Some would call it blessing,
   a quick, merciful end
   for one whose time has come.
   Thus I console myself:
   the best death is swift and painless.

Why then do I see myself
   carelessly cutting the slender-threaded rope
   by which he clung to life?
   His fall was silent.
   It was I who screamed:
   "Not my doing!"
But no reassuring voice
   whispers, consoling,
   "No, not you."

I forget sometimes
   the cost of entering that frail shell
   that cradles men.
I intervene with peril:
      at my risk, and theirs.
   No matter that I intend only good;
   all I do for healing's sake
   still holds the chance of harm.

That is the dark side
   to even the greatest enterprise.
And when the unbidden comes,
   the worst mistake
   is to pretend to be untouched.
To refuse the sight
   of one's dark failure
   condemns another,
   for naught forbids
   the same mistake again.
Let me not shield myself from pain.
   Let me see with clearer eyes
      my fallibility:
      I tried to heal you
      but lost instead.
      And I will fail again
         though much I wish it otherwise;
         human, as I am.
      Give me no pedestal
         from which to hang myself.
      It's pride that says never fail,
         must perfectly perform
         as if I were God, or god;
         as though not frail and faltering.
         Destined to fall short once and again,
         even as I seek to heal.

               Anne Egbert, MD

Confluence at Life's Extremes
David A. Silverman, MD, PhD

$\mathcal{I}$ spent last winter in the Neonatal Intensive Care Unit (NICU). This was a radical change from my usual venue, where the average patient is 86 years of age and the typical child past menopause. Although I am a faculty member, because I am a geriatrician my privileges in the NICU were defined by parenthood. Delivery of our first child was precipitated by placental abruptio, after a gestation too brief for Sarah Beth to survive without the expertise of physicians, the risks of high technology, and the mercy of something I don't quite believe in. One cannot grow from fertilized egg to free-living baby girl in just 28 weeks without singular help, substantial resources, and a bit of luck. She was 2 pounds, 4 ounces at birth and at her smallest weighed 1 pound, 13 ounces. We were warned that she would probably need mechanical ventilation and, barring complications, she'd be in the hospital about 3 months. And the list of complications? It was long and potent, even without the respiratory syncytial virus that went around that spring, killing two of her comrades. I was nearly driven mad by the bells and buzzers in the NICU. I nearly drove the neonatologists mad by seeing and comprehending too much and too little. When there was a moment to talk, they wondered aloud about this odd Beast, the geriatrician, for whom there seemed to be no Beauty.

"When we win," I was told, "we get 80 years of life. What do you get?"

"A moment of comfort; a treatable disorder revealed; a fracture prevented; an hour of dignity; a week or decade of improved function; a well-lived life repaid; a 70-year-old child at ease with a parent's care; a sensible death, safe from intensive care units for bigger people."

Everything was not always said aloud.

"If you lose, you get a dead baby, or a handicapped one, or parents beating their breasts in torment."

"If you lose," they thought, "does anyone give a damn?"

"The person whose burden of illness has not been eased will know."

Still, we had common interests. Neurologic function was one. The importance of the brain's well-being never diminishes with age. Neonatologists are rightfully attentive to its status. (Enough oxygen? Too much oxygen?) Then, for most of us, the welfare of the brain is a nonissue until we fall into the hands of geriatricians, in whose patient population brain failure provides abundant stereotypes.

Neonatologists and geriatricians are also especially attentive to the gastrointestinal tract. Our tiny girl needed to grow and mature enough for her gut to work and to gain adequate strength for eating. Enteral feedings started at 12 calories per day and progressed slowly. We endured two radiographs to look for a "nec," as the intern called necrotizing enterocolitis. Sarah Beth was never cursed with that malady, but we saw its monstrous effects in her peers. Elimination was also an issue. For a while she was dependent on 0.5-cc enemas. At the nursing home, gastrointestinal function, related both to feeding and defecation, if unsuitably dealt with, is also emotionally and physically costly as well as potentially lethal.

I thought that the infant across the aisle had a bad pressure sore on her buttocks. At last, something with which I was familiar. However, the look-alike was a giant hemangioma that had undergone painful necrosis. Treatment at that stage was not dissimilar from that rendered the unfortunately more common geriatric consequence of compromised capillaries.

Other parallel themes were also braided together: surrogates, ethics, hope, abandonment, and courage. They never visited or perhaps they visited too much. Whose best interests did they have in mind? They really loved their parent or child, even though they were so different from what they were or will become. Who is going to pay for all this?

The neonatologist and the geriatrician were unlocked momentarily from the extremes of existence, where the problem of life begins and where the solution is seen with its end. The life barely begun and the life nearly done bond physicians who seem at first to be far apart, but who in fact can easily touch because life traces a circle, bringing into proximity its beginning and its end. The geriatrician is familiar with death coming after a long life. Part of the job is to get it done right. Death is no stranger to the neonatologist either, although it is oddly different after a short life.

Sarah Beth did well. She was never artificially ventilated, had no ventricular bleeding, no sepsis, no necrotizing enterocolitis, no lung disease, no brain disease. She was the tiniest and most precious being in the world, and she kept her parents running scared for 3 months. Now she's big; she laughs and talks and thoroughly enjoys the world. So hard to think of her as ever getting old, so hard to think of a woman named Sarah who died yesterday as ever having been young.

Christmas on the AIDS Ward

Lazarus died and Jesus wept.
—John 11

When AIDS patients try to talk
and are near death
the former Surgeon General said
they are like kittens.
They open their mouths to cry
but no sound comes out.

The virus spreads
even on holy days.
It replicates even during feasts.
It robs us of strength
even on most high and holy days.

But on the AIDS ward
during Christmas there is
strength and reason
enough to weep.

David L. Schiedermayer, MD

Vespers

Come, night, at morning skilled hands cut this wrist,
Alter channels that blood once racing pure,
Now unclean, in arterial floods enter
Veins, pound, stretch them, thicken walls that bulge, twist

To ripe blood sausages needle points burst,
Let quick blood run out, be laved, return pure,
Reeking of machine. Manacle, sign, scar,
Pain's badge, my mark unto the final rest,

Let me hide from you in one last sweet dream,
Remember fingers petaled on this stalk
Ringed in amulets, cuffed in Venice lace,

Held high in dance to catch a candle's gleam;
My love, take my hand now in your warm touch,
Grace what I must sacrifice with your kiss.

Fred Coe, MD

The Miracle of the Eye
Ralph E. Yodaiken, MD, MPH

Light strikes the retina, activating photoreceptor rods and cones. Immediately, impulses discharge through a myriad of bipolar and ganglion cells, along fibers that gather in bundles of optic nerves and stream like two converging rivers to the chiasma, spreading from there to junctions beneath the brain. Here at the geniculate body, colors are sorted—blues, reds, and greens. From these junctions nerve fibers course to the visual cortex at the back of the brain for processing shape and form—flowers, grass, sky. The need for action blends with stored experience, the interpretive melding almost instantaneously. Move forward to smell, smile, proceed with caution, whatever it takes for motion or stillness, flight or rest. The eye, a complex machine beyond comprehension, has evolved through eons of hunger, hunt, fear, and survival.

Wiped out by a single bullet—rods and cones, branching neural connections, chemical end points. Capillary channels fill with coagulating plasma and stagnant, anoxic red cells. Ten-year-old eyes glazed, not by age or disease, cataracts or thrombosis, but by a round, metal projectile smashing through the skull or heart, shutting down the magnificent machines, forever. Presidents of the United States and members of Congress deem bullet and gun indispensable to the defense of the people, by the people, against the people. This, too, is the judgment of the President of the National Rifle Association.

The child standing at the street lamp views his world; cars, buses, and people stream by.

C A R.

Car. Careful, careful comes the caution from the cortical cells. Do not step off the pavement. Stored images of mother and teacher, wagging fingers. No, do not! The eyes absorb the curbstones, the feet stay put; tires sweep by. Mother and teacher will be pleased. The lips spread in a smile as the metal bullet intended for someone or no one, smashes through the skull. The child's eye machines gel. No more messages to the feet. No more tears flowing from the lacrimal glands to the puncta lacrimalia and into the ducts. The transparent corneas no longer need moisture. They dull in accordance with the laws of the land, of Presidents and the intent of Congress. In death the lenses behind each cornea swell.

There are 10 layers of cells in the retina, 7 million color-sensitive cones, and 100 million light-sensitive rods. Bipolar neurons stretch from the rods and cones to the ganglion cells. Light sprayed with dark shadows from the streets of Washington, D.C., capital of the United States, passes through each lens to the retinas.

A 19-year-old man is fatally shot in S.E. Washington. The pupil, the aperture of the eye, restricts the amount of light passing through the lens. In the dark, the pupils dilate to allow the rods as much light as possible at 3:15 a.m. But the pupils also dilate because of fear, and pain, so the tense 19-year-old's pupils are dilated as widely as possible in the murky shadows, from fear and then, suddenly, from pain. At that very moment, in the early hours of the morning, with the nation at peace, the eyes of the sleeping Presidents are covered by eyelids, necessary to prevent desiccation. The surfaces of living eyes must always remain moist.

When will the first of the summer-weekend shooting deaths occur this year? Maybe on Friday at 10:55 p.m. as happened last year when police found a 26-year-old who later died in the hospital. Early Saturday morning, last year, after daybreak, police said a dispute resulted in gunfire. A young male from Ninth Street N.W. was shot several times. No one was arrested. At 3:00 p.m., Saturday, police responded to a reported shooting in S.E. Washington. This time, a Hispanic man was pronounced dead at the D.C. General Hospital. He was 48 years old and died of gunshot wounds. Early Sunday morning during a concert in Congress Heights, one teenager was shot dead and three others were wounded. An arrest was made, last year.

Light entering the eye is bent at four surfaces, at each surface of the cornea and at each surface of the lens, to converge on the retina and project an inverted image. Fibers pull on the elastic capsule of the lens to accommodate the image. The near point of accommodation, the closest point an object can be brought to the eye without distortion, must have been about 10 cm for the youngest of those shot dead in Washington.

Between 16 and 20 cm for the 48-year-old Hispanic man.

With age the lens hardens. Adjustments become more difficult. As the President ages he will not be able to read a book at 40 cm. True now for the other President—the one who heads the National Rifle Association. Older eyes require presbyopic correction by a convex lens. The frames fit snugly over the nose. Those other citizens, the ones dying in the streets of Washington D.C., won't be bothered by that expense.

The President of the United States, the most powerful democracy in the world, requires global vision. Nearer to home, however, his vision is more restricted. The past President of the United States was an avid golfer. His weak point was putting. He had a putting green built on the grounds of the White House. The image cast on the two retinas is two-dimensional. Positioning the three-dimensional golf ball and estimating the length it has to travel requires depth perception. To putt the ball he looks toward the hole. The lenses accommodate. Cortical cells compare the two images emanating from the eyes and estimate the distance to the hole. The putter moves back, then swiftly forward. The ball rolls into the hole. The new President jogs around the new White House jogging track set up just for him. He needs only to judge distance correctly. President Clinton's eyes take in the smiling reporters. He smiles.

A well-regulated Militia being necessary to the security of a Free State, the right of the people to keep and bear arms shall not be infringed.

Cells similar to the "near" and "far" cells of the cat are very sensitive to distances. These are called "disparity" cells, and they respond to stationary or moving stimuli at variable distances. For example, a 46-year-old man was killed and three young children were shot and wounded when a man in a car fired into a crowd of people in the 1300 block of Park Road N.W. The wounded were two girls, 7 and 11 years old, and a 4-year-old boy. The gunman fired the shots from a dark-colored car that sped away. Stimuli from the targets were coordinated and lined up instantly by disparity cells of the gunner in the dark moving car.

"Blood was pouring out of the girl's neck," said a man who ran to the scene. Poor man. Messages from the awkward, twisted shapes sped through the rapidly accommodating lenses as he came closer and closer to the bright red blood.

This year the disturbed mind in the Mount Pleasant area used a shotgun. He killed two persons and wounded several others. Perhaps the relatively poor shots, the unplanned survival of some targets, were related to what is known as stereoblindness, an inability to judge depth or distance correctly. The condition is relatively common, particularly when strabismus, failure of the eyes to work in parallel, goes undetected.

Even closing the eyes for prolonged periods does not result in permanent blindness. Thus, members of Congress can close their eyes for an entire Congressional session and not go blind, provided they remain alive and all body systems continue to function. When they ultimately lift their lids, all visual acuity is recovered within a short time. They can, in other words, go on with their games without losing any of the benefits of the protracted sleep.

To Respond Always
Douglas R. Mailman, MD

$\mathcal{M}$ay 30th . . . graduation day at last. The ceremony was moved inside at the last minute because of rain. The exercises began with the speaker's suggestion to find a niche in medicine for which we had a passion. Her passion for her own work was evident, encouraging. The candidates were presented. We became doctors, our degree stating, ". . . with all the rights, privileges and honors, as well as the obligations and responsibilities . . . ."

"Responsibilities" grabbed me. While we were reciting the Physician's Oath, I heard it again: "to respond always." Benediction . . . recessional . . . then the search through the crowd to find my family. After accepting their congratulations, my wife and I excused ourselves to pick up our young children from a friend's house. On the way, we were talking about the events of the evening when we passed several stopped vehicles. My wife said, "Someone's down!"

I ran to the scene to find a young Asian man face down in the street. He wore no shirt, no shoes, and blood was everywhere. His only movement was a slight rhythmic head nod; he silently gasped for air. The people standing around did nothing but stare. I knelt beside him; there was no pulse, no respiration.

Instinctively, I knew what to do. I asked for help. The only response was, "Don't move him." Although it felt strange, I said, "I'm a doctor." While turning him over, I was nauseated by the smell of stale beer and fresh blood.

ABCs.

His jaw was shattered. I removed several teeth while attempting to clear his airway. I wiped as much of the blood from his mouth and face as I could. I knew the next step was to establish breathing, but I had no mask.

Blood. AIDS. Hepatitis.

I recalled the lifesaving instructor at Boy Scout camp saying, "When saving a life, the most important life is your own." I stared at this man, knowing that mouth-to-mouth was his only chance. Again I wiped his face, but blood still oozed from his mouth.

I was relieved when the emergency medical service arrived soon after. They began cardiopulmonary resuscitation with gloved hands and a bag-mask. They quickly loaded him into the ambulance and were working on him while I watched. Feeling helpless and confused, I got back in my car and wiped my hands with every baby-wipe I could find. We left quietly to retrieve our children. On the way back, we passed the still blocked off area and I slowed, trying to see if the blood was still on the ground. The pavement had been washed by the steady drizzle. There was no sign of where that young man had fallen.

Over the next few days I struggled with my response to those events. Was I irresponsible in not starting mouth-to-mouth immediately? What if he had been dressed in coat and tie? Was I fulfilling the responsibility demanded of me? Was I upholding the Physician's Oath? I questioned my actions, sought the advice of more experienced physicians, and asked several people what they would have done.

I am still confused about what happened that night, but I do know a little more about what responsibility means. That young man lay dying in the middle of the street and I had stopped. Although I had been trained for emergencies, that became superfluous in the events of that night. I had routinely helped resuscitate trauma victims in the emergency room of Parkland Memorial Hospital. In the middle of a wet street, kneeling in the blood of a dying man, I felt what responsibility means. I have spent many hours trying to put into words the tumult of emotions I experienced while caring for my first patient as a doctor. I can say that caring for people no longer seems routine. I also believe that responsibility has much to do with living the Physician's Oath, which states in part "to approach each patient with integrity, candor, empathy and respect" and "to remain conscious of my limitations."

This was quite a beginning, especially after taking "responsibility" so seriously. I am a doctor; that seems to be the easy part. Becoming a physician and living the Oath is the real challenge. While our commencement speaker encouraged us to find something worthwhile for which we had a passion, I had wondered if I would find mine. I believe I have.

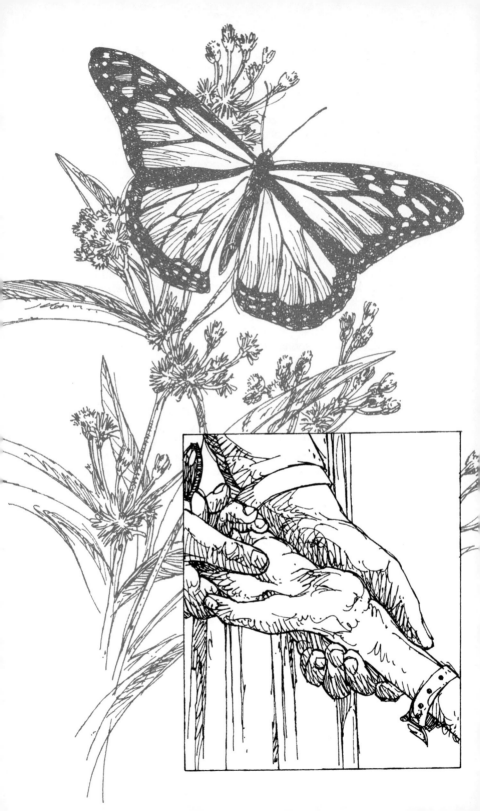

THEY FIND DOCTORS GOOD AND BAD AND SEARCH FOR A MENTOR

If the physician possess native sagacity, and a nameless something more—let us call it intuition; if he show no intrusive egotism, nor disagreeably prominent characteristics of his own; if he have the power, which must be born in him, to bring his mind into such affinity with his patient's, . . . then, at some inevitable moment, will the soul of the sufferer be dissolved, and flow forth in a dark, but transparent stream, bringing all its mysteries into the daylight.

Nathaniel Hawthorne

Fellows for Cons

It's never easy, knowing what to choose,
especially in a light rain. Should you lose
a stroke by chipping to the fairway? Should you drive
on through the trees? We'll both arrive
eventually, beginners always, though we've played
from Spring to Fall with rented clubs.
Your shameless Frosty the Snowman dance
has lost effect. It's almost chance,
your choosing in the woods, but be prepared
to duck in case your choosing fires back
against the trees to rattle like a pinball on
its bumpers. Our discussion by the pond
ripples with the woman from Vermont you call
each night. I watch you fall in love
with my Chicago skyline. Mallards play,
procrastinate, while we go back and forth:
practice or research, money or mankind,
kids or career. In refuge from
the ritualistic beating it endures,
we find your Spaulding 2, an egg
within a nest of pale blue butterwort
beside a row of elderbush, the seeds of which
are spread with birds that eat their fruit.
By muffling rain, the woodland hooch
allows the birdfoot violet voice:
you will not linger long with me
among the oak, azalea, wisteria and nameless
other underbrush. Monsieur Frostaceous, shameless
in his taunting, will achieve. You know
I favor chipping from the woods
and getting safely into play, for happiness
is dog-legged to the left. Or right. Your guess
is as good as mine. I can see you now,
the itinerant pro, playing the great courses
of Bethesda, Boston, over wide-raked traps
with every slash, every uncock of the wrists,
hoping for daylight and bit hitting down
narrow and fast-running fairways.

Phillip J. Cozzi, MD

Are We Always? When Do We Stop?

H. J. Van Peenen, MD

Dysart, Christian, M.D., License #7265 (Salem, Marion County, Oregon)

The board and the physician entered into a Retired Status Agreement without Findings and Order. The effective date of retirement was January 1, 1992. RETIRED STATUS AGREEMENT WITHOUT FINDINGS AND ORDER SIGNED: December 27, 1991

That is the exact wording in the *Bulletin* of the Medical Disciplinary Board of the Board of Medical Examiners of a neighboring state. It comes to me four times a year.

But Chris Dysart is not just another name in the *Bulletin*. He is a long-standing friend. We have shown each other slides of our journeys into the Karakorums or the Galapagos, squired each other's wives to the country club, even taken a cruise together. And in his Christmas card, which announced his impending retirement, he had said nothing of the reasons for it.

That was his privilege, of course, but inevitably I had to wonder what he had done to earn his sanction. I hoped that it was only because he had become physically or mentally unable to handle his work. Still, I knew from reading the *Bulletin* over the years that there were only a few ways a physician could lose his license, and gross incompetence was rarely one of them. And I also knew that Chris was not too impaired to practice. Like most of us he had had a bypass, but his mind was as alert as ever; he was still in the category of "young-old"; and in a recent conversation he had denounced my own early retirement as a cop-out, proclaiming his intention to hang on for at least another 5 years.

I was and am in no position to determine my friend's competence to practice his specialty for we are social friends only. We have never worked in the same hospital, referred patients to each other, or asked each other for advice on the phone. But I have to assume from his obvious success that he was thought competent by referring physicians and agencies. With considerable regret, I moved on to the more common indications for sanction.

The *Bulletin* had taught me that most physicians who are disciplined seem to have been so for either personal substance abuse, a sexual offense, or Medicare fraud. Knowing Chris as I did, knowing the strength of his marriage and his lifetime abstinence from drugs and alcohol, it seemed the only one of the usual charges that might fit was fraud, abuse not of patients but of the governmental agency that rules our lives. But he hadn't told me that; it would be discourteous to ask, and so I will never know. Yet I will do him the disservice—and probably the injustice—of wondering for the rest of my life.

That led me to ponder how I should behave toward a colleague who has been sanctioned. Although I have no problem accepting someone who has been convicted of fraud by the rather dubious standards of Medicare auditors, I must, of course, excommunicate from professional contact someone who has been guilty of abusing a patient. But what about the addict, no longer fit to practice medicine, who is perhaps as much a victim as criminal? Do you address him as "Doctor"? Is it proper to discuss cases with him or fill up the conversation with gossip about reimbursement policies and denials by PSROs? May I take him to a party sponsored by Devon Pharmaceuticals? In other words, is he, although sanctioned, still one of us? Sometimes he is, I think, but the line for that decision is fine.

I am told that a defrocked priest, forbidden to administer the sacraments, is still a priest, that the ordination cannot be undone even by the Pope. Perhaps that is also true of a sanctioned physician, especially if all he has done has been to run afoul of some minor regulation enforced by a third-rate bureaucrat. Or misinterpreted a fee directive. Or been falsely denounced by a deranged or vindictive patient.

In the case of Chris such musings will not matter. We are social friends only, and I will treat him as I always have, but sooner or later the same sanction could be imposed on someone to whom I once referred a patient or from whom I received referrals. Would I stop talking medicine to a former colleague who had lost his license? Probably not, but our talk might lose much of its meaning.

One thought leads by leaps and bounds to unrelated issues. I began to wonder if we weren't all sanctioned ultimately by time, fading powers, obsolete knowledge, the inevitable drifting away of patients, and diminution in status that comes with simple old age. At what stage in our careers do we cease to be doctors and become undeserving of the honorific "MD" after our names?

Perhaps guidance could come from those who took the degree but never practiced. When do we become doctors in the first place? Are Somerset Maugham, Armand Hammer, Michael Crichton, part of our guild? Obviously, Armand Hammer thought he was for he used the honorific for nearly 70 years. But Maugham seems never to have referred to himself as "Dr." nor does Michael Crichton. They lived and live as literary men. Justly so. Medical authors who practice medicine, Lewis Thomas, John Stone, Perri Klass, Richard Selzer, William Ober, Gerald Weissman, always seem to be proudly doctors first. I believe it is the actual contact with patients and colleagues that makes us see ourselves as doctors and not as writers or business persons. It is active medical work that makes us members of the guild.

So, more to the point then, is do we cease being doctors when we no longer see patients? When should we stop expecting from others the special respect an active doctor is usually granted?

For some the answer is "never"! Dr. Glass insisted on the privilege until he died. When I practiced in Iowa, he was the only physician in a small neighboring town who, at age 85, finally gave up his last few, very loyal, elderly patients. He was an honorable man who had always practiced within his limitations and maintained the affection of his peers until the day he died. But by the time I knew him he had gone from being a busy, competent, useful physician to a trembling old man, far gone in dementia. He lived in a chair at the nursing home, his withered hands holding an *AMA News* he could no longer read or understand. Yet even in the home, he was not "Jim" or "Bill" like the other patients; he was "Dr. Glass" until he died in his sleep, and he is "Dr. Glass" still, for his tombstone proudly portrays "MD" after his name.

Many of us are different from Dr. Glass. We retire young and build another identity so we need not cling to our status, need not insist on being greeted as "Dr." wherever we move. In fact, for those of us who spend our time away from practice on a retirement hobby, a second career, on managing investments, on being the beloved patriarch of a growing family, the appellation, "MD," becomes irrelevant. More and more I find myself leaving it off when I type a signature line or a return address. Yet, there are still moments when I want to be a doctor, accepted as such by my contemporaries, and granted the respect the young guildsman should have for his elder. I reserve the right to dress in that elegant, but understated way we have inherited. If invited to walk in an academic procession, I would still proudly wear the three green stripes on my sleeve and the doctoral hood of my alma mater. But I am not really a doctor any more. I do not practice. I have given up my licenses before they could be taken from me. And perhaps, in the eyes of some, my insistence on "MD" for the tombstone makes me as much a fraud as my friend, Chris, disciplined, presumably, for overbilling.

La Cuenta*

John P. Bramante, MD

*C*uentame [Tell me]," he said, and she did.

She sat across from him. I sat to the side. She was 19 years old with long black frizzy hair, a sharp pointed nose, and thin painted lips. Her face betrayed the bony ridges and the labyrinth of cartilage that lay beneath. With the suppleness of youth, her floating skin was still smooth and her smile was wide and wild. She was tall for a Mapuche and her young breasts defined a proud figure beneath her one-size-too-small V-neck sweater.

"Nineteen days," he said, "How did that number arrive? When was your last bleeding?"

"In January . . . January 29th."

He sat across the desk and stared at her. He had vivid blue eyes. There, in that South American countryside of short dark native people, his blue eyes were remarkable—they reflected the German blood of my Maestro. He sat, staring, and she clarified.

"The next time should have been February 28th and that makes 19 days," she said slowly, poised.

"Your last time of bleeding was January 29th—with nothing in between?"

"Yes, Doctor."

"That makes you 3 weeks late, more or less."

"Yes, Doctor."

"In a year, how many times are you late?"

"Never, Doctor."

"You have never been late?" he asked incredulously.

"No, Doctor."

He continued to stare in silence, never taking his eyes from her. Finally, he said, "Show me your hands."

She put them on the desk, palms down. She continued to smile.

"Turn them over," he said, while he took them himself and turned them over so that they lay supine in front of him. Surprisingly, he did not take the wrist between his thumb and middle finger as he usually did. Instead, he sat with his hands folded in front of him and inspected the soft, dark, dirty hands while they waited there to be

---

Cuenta: a narrative or report; also a bill or the cost.

told what to do. He said to her, "Take off your sweater and lie down," and then to me, "Please examine this woman's heart."

She did not hesitate to move. This visit was to be her moment of glory, verifying her great accomplishment. The Doctor wrote. While she undressed, I asked about her relations. She turned and said with modest playfulness, "I'm married," using the permanent form of the verb "to be." I had looked for a ring on her finger but of course she was not wearing one.

She had the type of heart murmur that comes from a narrowing of the outlet valve of the heart. The blood roared through this valve and the sound followed the rush of blood into the young woman's neck. But her pulse did not coincide. Instead of being weak and drawn out as in pure valve narrowing, it was sharp and transient. It was the pulse of a valve that does not close correctly, that allows blood to fall back into the heart. When I finished my examination, the Doctor listened carefully to her heart and neck, felt her pulse, and returned to his seat and continued his writing.

Finally, he turned his eyes to me and asked me what I thought. I explained what I had heard and the discrepant pulse and I offered my tentative diagnosis.

"Exactly," he said in English, the language he sometimes chose when speaking with me. Turning back again and looking at her, he said, "She has both aortic stenosis and insufficiency . . . but it is not so strange, they often occur together. This is probably from the infection. The mitral valve was clean to me." I nodded and he asked what I thought of the diastolic murmur.

"I didn't hear it," I said after a moment.

"Neither did I," he said in Spanish while he wrote, "but it is probably there. What thing told me she has an anormalidad?"

"The devil," I thought, but did not dare say. Many times he had shown a Faustian genius for observing physical characteristics but an insensitivity toward the less tangible of his patients' concerns.

"I don't know," I replied.

"What about this woman's body is urging us to examine her heart?" he asked with a patience that demanded an intelligent answer. Her face had changed to one that was stubborn about its happiness. "What tells you she has a defect?" he asked again, a little louder.

It had been there before, I had seen it before. "The pulsation in her sternal notch," I said.

"Perfecto. That pulse is not normal." He said this looking straight into me with those piercing blue eyes. "Never forget this. Your senses: Your eyes, your fingers, your ears and nose are finer than all the machines you will use. That is the truth." I made no reply.

He ripped the pink slip from the pad he had been writing on and offered it over the desk. He said to her, "I agree, you are probably pregnant. But there is a problem with your heart. It might be bad, it might not be. I doubt it will hurt your baby. I want it to be looked at by a specialist. Take that paper and have them make you an appointment in Temuco, then make an appointment to start your visits. Do you understand me?"

"Yes, Doctor," she said in the tone of a scolded school child. She stood up and carefully pushed the chair back into place.

"Listo [Ready]," he said.

"Ciao," she replied, her back to us as she left.

To Oxford

Yellow roses on stately stone walls
venerable ivy in venerable crevices
walking by the Thames gives a vista of the town
nearly the same now
so I am told
as known by generations of scholars before
how peaceful are the ducks
how close is God here
in the grass
tiny farmhouses
sunset glowing over a field
No wonder I became so soon fond

How far is God here
from an eight by ten room in the hospital
with a phone and a pager
on one side a laboratory crammed to the rafters
on the other a room
where I have recently stood gowned
gloved up to the elbow
in someone else's blood
How earnestly I long for ducks
and grass and ivy
and crevices and courtyards
or courage.

Martha Harwit, MD

The ER Incident

Terry Eli Hill, MD

The Uncertainty of Housestaff

*D*isputes about the incident flourished throughout the hospital for months. The personalities of those involved quickly became less important than the race and group they represented. Simplifying failed to clarify, however, and discussions about race, in particular, were awkward and inconclusive.

The housestaff were of multiple races and backgrounds. For most, choosing to train in an inner city public hospital reflected what we thought was a deep sense of purpose. Our feelings about being physicians were to grow more complex, however, not least because the community's unresolved problems battered and wearied us. The ER incident eventually came to embody that complexity of purpose, that uncertainty about where we stood and who we served.

The Incident

The emergency department was having a retirement party in the suburbs for its outgoing chief. The chief had become frankly cynical, a frequent user of terms like "dirtball." Two of my fellow residents and several nurses thought it would be fitting to bring a surprise guest, one of the emergency room "regulars." The regular who happened to be available was a homeless alcoholic who often spent days in successive ER evaluations separated by brief intervals outside, usually brought in by the police for belligerence or stupor, usually diagnosed as post-ictal or just plain drunk.

He agreed to come to the party and seemed pleased when the staff cleaned him up, cut his hair, and dressed him. On the ride out with one of the residents, he talked about his youth, family, and disappointments, surprising the resident with some degree of clarity and insight. Once at the house he had misgivings, however, and would not go in. The involved staff kept him company for a few hours, bringing him food and drink, then took him back to the hospital.

The patient was black. The staff members involved were white.

Two weeks later, when the incident became known, charges of racism and hate made banner headlines.

The Not-So-Distant Past

In 1963, an anthropologist began his research in the hospital and later published the following observations:

> Doctors frequently talk negatively of the facilities and the patient population, not so much to indicate a desire for change . . . as to maintain a social distance from implicit identification with "this kind of medicine" and "this kind of patient."

The practice developed in the Emergency Unit several years ago of keeping an informal digest of "funny" instances of Negro folk medicine knowledge and vocabularies . . . . The dozen-or-so-page list is hung on the bulletin board in the doctors' office and is periodically consulted, during slack work hours, as a source of humor. It contains such references as "I's got a sore in my bagi-va," "My die Betsies is acting up," "I's had venal disease," etc. . . .

Derogatory talk about patients is rather common, particularly about those patients whose behavior, way of life, when regarded from a middle-class per-spective, are considered morally obnoxious.

I had discovered this work by accident in a used bookstore in a dis-tant city. When I read this passage to a conference of housestaff and attendings after the ER incident, the room became absolutely still. No one had known about the study. No one had heard stories about the list of "funny Negro sayings."

Many of us had chosen the hospital because of its current reputa-tion for service and advocacy. We had no idea that its history was so troublesome or so close.

Aftermath

For days the press printed charges that the intent in the ER incident was to ridicule the patient, consistent with a pattern of racial ten-sions at the hospital. Someone from the black community remem-bered an incident from years past in which her relative—his hypo-glycemia undiagnosed—was tossed out of the emergency room as a "nigger drunk." Hospital administrators publicly announced their intent to discipline those involved.

The two doctors were stunned. They had been seen by others and themselves as caring and diligent physicians. The irony they had intended was directed toward their retiring chief, not at the patient.

The patient himself was delighted with the attention. His visits con-tinued uninterrupted. As before, the social workers' many attempts to help were stymied by a lack of resources and the patient's own intransigence.

The housestaff argued about everything. We argued about the facts. We argued whether the incident was racist, and if so, was the racism more or less important than our prejudice against people without jobs, homes, or education. We argued whether we as a group shared any responsibility. We argued whether we should publicly acknowl-edge that racism continued to exist in our hospital.

And we circled our wagons: The hospital is cynically underfunded, we said. The impropriety of an isolated incident pales before the daily, relentless dehumanization of both patients and staff, the grotesque mismatch between needs and resources. We said, finally, to some of our critics who seemed ill-informed or high-handed: If you don't work in our ER, keep your righteousness to yourself.

History

The hospital occasionally made the national news for its afflictions of trauma and crack, poverty and underfunding. So I was only a little surprised, during a visit to my parents' home in their small southern town, to hear them ask how our celebrated patient was doing.

I was more surprised during this same visit when I read an old rendering of our family history. The account begins with an Irish immigrant who fought in the Revolutionary War, notes church and civic contributions, then makes this statement about my great-great-great grandfather: "Besides a large body of land he owned 103 slaves at his death in 1843." The family prosperity faded shortly thereafter. My generation is largely unaware of that land, those slaves.

Although this discovery and the ER incident became linked in my own mind, I didn't mention it on my return to the hospital. Even in relaxed settings, our mixed-group discussions about race had been impersonal and circumspect. But beyond my personal connection, can remembering slavery offer any insight into the incident?

The concept of racism is necessary but far from sufficient to explain either the ER incident or the havoc of broken lives that we spend so much time patching up in emergency rooms. Class and lifestyle differences separate us from our patients more consistently than race. But remembering white attitudes toward black slaves can help illustrate the danger that housestaff face in confronting this havoc. Regardless of the race of the patient or the house officer, there is a tendency to see "this kind of patient" as "morally obnoxious," less than fully human. This sense of moral superiority is a moral flaw for house officers as much as it was for slave owners. Its embodiment is cynicism.

The Challenge of Recognition

In his study of a British general practitioner, John Berger described the cultural gulfs between this physician and the uneducated villagers he served, as well as the patience and initiative required to achieve intimacy with them.

Initially enamored of emergencies and dramatic surgeries, this doctor, over the years, shifted his keenest interest from diagnosis and treatment to the doctor-patient relationship. Increasingly aware and accepting of his own weaknesses, he looked across the divisions of education and culture for the similarities between his patients and himself. Gradually he began to sense that knowledge of the villagers was a kind of self-knowledge, that the structure of their stories was also the structure of his. Over time, his patients responded. They came to regard him as a good doctor not because of his technical competence, which they took for granted: "No, he is acknowledged as a good doctor because he meets the deep but unformulated expectation of the sick for a sense of fraternity. He recognizes them."

The Uncertainty of Human Value

Is it fair to impose a country practitioner's ideal of connectedness on inner city emergency physicians? The emergency room is among the most depersonalized of patient care settings. In the absence of personal connectedness, what motivates good medicine there is professionalism: the challenge of getting the right diagnosis, applying the right treatment. The ethic of respect for the patient within professionalism, however, is more superficial than within the country practitioner's ideal. It failed to prevent the impropriety of our residents in an act that would have been unthinkable for Berger's physician.

Berger concludes, "One of the fundamental reasons why so many doctors become cynical and disillusioned is precisely because, when the abstract idealism has worn thin, they are uncertain about the value of the actual lives of the patients they are treating."

Our Constitution set the reckoning of slaves at three-fifths human. In our society today money provides the most common and convenient measurement of human value. The poor themselves are further divided into "deserving" and "undeserving," and the latter are often disproportionately black. Amidst this uncertainty of human value, incidents like the one in our emergency room are predictable.

Now that my residency is done, I wonder if my own cynicism has already grown too large. Perhaps an awareness of my personal flaws can help me beyond the obvious differences toward "recognition" of my patients, as Berger says, and compassion for the reluctant players in this particular history.

A Navajo Sabbatical

When I first came
to the Navajo reservation
I was afraid of heights
I was afraid of horses running free
I could not walk the canyon rim
(too much flatland in my past).

But now I like to dance
if only
back here in the midwest
if only
before clinic in the morning.

And now I remember
when I look at the moon
a Navajo man who lived
by Coalmine Canyon
and rode his horse every day
across the high desert.

And now I hear
his high voice singing
when the geese rise
from the pond by the hospital asphalt.

And now I recall
climbing Castle Rock to the very top.

I gave the Navajos
only some doctoring
but they gave me new rest
new courage
new strength
and a poem to remember
by an unknown Navajo poet:

"Today we are blessed with a beautiful baby.
May his feet be to the east
May his right hand be to the south
May his head be to the west
May his left hand be to the north.
May he walk and dwell on mother earth peacefully.
May he be blessed with assorted soft valued goods.
May he be blessed with precious variegated stones.
May he be blessed with fat sheep in variation.
I ask these blessings with reverence and holiness
May mother, the earth, the sky, the sun, the moon together
my father
May the essence of life be old age.
May the source of happiness be beauty.
All in peace, all in beauty,
all in harmony
all in happiness."

David L. Schiedermayer, MD

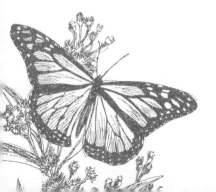

Intuition of a Clinical Sort
Herbert J. Keating III, MD

Taking care of doctors can often teach us how to take better care of other patients, especially when a given doctor-patient is a clinician of the highest excellence. I must tell you about Dr. John. I always looked forward to his visits. As the retired dean of pediatrics, John had seen it all in medicine. He began his practice when physicians were more revered than now, during an era when a baby who was not meant to survive did not. Grief was often eased by a doctor's contribution to a collective certainty that God's will had been done. Dr. John was present for the introduction of medical miracles, like penicillin and heart surgery, at a time when only physicians could command the magical science of it all. Every encounter I had with him taught me something. His lessons were delivered modestly and in parable form; sometimes I didn't appreciate them until much later, when the pressures of office hours were replaced by contemplation. I remember one afternoon especially well.

Dr. John looked dapper as usual, although a recent bout of pneumonia had made him thinner. His white hair was slicked back precisely, and his mustache was well trimmed. I asked him the usual questions about relevant symptoms and then invited him up onto the examination table.

"You don't need me to get completely undressed, Bert, do you?" John asked. His speech was clipped and precise, delivered in a voice made hoarse by decades of talking loudly to parents above the cries of their wailing children.

"Just listen to my heart and lungs," he instructed, and then slowly ascended onto the table, tugging off his tie and unbuttoning his immaculately ironed shirt. "You don't need to poke me anywhere else today, do you?"

Shirtless, leaning forward on the edge of the table, he volunteered his bony chest toward my stethoscope, and I listened. I told him he sounded fine and that I didn't want to change any of his medications. I said that I did want to obtain another chest x-ray.

"Fine, fine," he pronounced. As he pushed himself off the table to a standing position he asked, "Did I ever tell you the story about the refrigerator in the nursery?"

Listening for my response, John cocked his right ear forward with his hand, which made a flesh-colored hearing aid more obvious.

"Don't think so, John."

"Damnedest thing, really, Bert. I was working at the St. Francis, in their six-bed newborn nursery, and instead of one of the beds they had installed this refrigerator. Right in the middle of the place!

173

Awful thing, but they needed to keep the formula refrigerated, and they had nowhere else to put it.

"This refrigerator made the most horrible racket. Like a bass drum, literally shaking the floor."

As he spoke, John got dressed, and he began to look natty again. He continued the story as if he were entertaining at a dinner party he was hosting.

"One late afternoon I was making rounds at the hospital. I remember this clearly, like it was yesterday. There was this baby girl, and I put my stethoscope on the child's back, and I couldn't hear a thing. I thought it was because of the racket from the icebox, and I stuffed my stethoscope in my pocket and announced to everyone within earshot, in a rather irritated fashion I might add, that I couldn't possibly practice pediatrics with a refrigerator in the room.

"I was full of myself then, Bert. I had done that stint in Boston, you know. I thought they should have jumped up and unplugged that refrigerator.

"Well, later that night I was lying in bed. It was very late, but I got this terrible feeling that something was wrong. I had no idea what, but I knew that I had to examine that baby again. So I got up and got dressed. My wife hardly stirred, she was so accustomed to me getting up at all hours. I went back into that nursery, and listened to that baby again. And do you know what I found?

"I found that I couldn't hear the baby's breath sounds all right, but just on the one side. Yes, the refrigerator was on, everything was the same, but I could hear sounds on the other side!

"It wasn't the refrigerator at all!" John said triumphantly. "The baby had a huge diaphragmatic hernia! I got the pediatric surgeon to see her, and he fixed her up right away."

John paused and then said clearly, "You see, Bert, somehow I got called back to that baby. What called me back?"

I was silent.

John added, hastily, "It's happened before, at other times, too. What do you suppose called me back that night, Bert?"

The question seemed too difficult at first, and I didn't answer him. John thought he was making me uncomfortable.

"Don't want to take up any more of your time, son," John said, and then he left me alone.

An Obvious Truth

Asked about tautologies, the tweedy prof,
Reflectively tapping his pipe on a worn-down heel,
Makes tenured utterance: "Birds are birds."

Just so, the past is well behind you
And while it is possible to repeat mistakes
There is, thankfully, no way to relive it.

Every day, then, must be a new beginning
With no allowance for who you were.
The weightiest prize yesterday could offer
Accentuates the blankness of this present page
While paunch, stoop and a sprinkling of hoar
Belie the campaigns, the victory, the parched hurrahs
That happened to someone whose scars are still yours.

A brave private can make an indecisive captain
And, no matter how retouched, the years
Refuse your overtures, those very ones
Emptied of all truth for now
That regale the bedtimes of an unbelieving child.

Joseph Herman, MD

Canary Cage and China

Covered with husks and wasted seeds
the drought field
unfolds in the corner,
beneath the canary cage
already the newspapers yellow.
The headlines say we're going to Mars,
while stealth and guns and crack
take the young in arms,
their bellies rife with parasites.
Yet one stands before tanks
and reaches toward knowledge
and water in the sand.
For the starving children
beyond the square
where the sun sets round,
stars turn to ash and fall
in waves like flags,
and the red blood runs
bright on broken bone china.

Joseph R. Thurn, MD

Parable of the Surgeon and the Internist
Susan N. Rosenthal, MD

As a medical oncologist with a special interest in breast cancer, I am frequently asked to see women after breast cancer surgery for consideration of systemic adjuvant therapy with tamoxifen, combination chemotherapy, or both. The patients are often under considerable psychological and emotional stress related to the recent diagnosis of cancer and the threat to body image that their recent surgery represents. The discussion I have with them involves complex issues such as the concept of micrometastatic disease, the statistical description of risk of recurrence in both absolute and relative terms, and the controversy over which is the best form of adjuvant therapy for the patient's disease stage, nodal status, menopausal status, and hormonal receptor status of her tumor. Clearly, at its best, this consultation is very difficult, lengthy, and troubling for the patient and any family members or friends who may accompany her. It is made considerably more difficult if the surgeon has already told the patient that she should receive tamoxifen and has prescribed it for her. Despite gentle hints that I would prefer to discuss these issues with the patient before any prescriptions for adjuvant therapy, I have been unable to change the practices of several of my referring surgeons in this regard. I have recently developed the following parable in an effort to produce an analogy that my surgical colleagues will understand.

Once upon a time there was an internist who took care of many female patients. He was very concerned about preventive measures, and he made sure that all of his patients had careful breast exams, were encouraged and instructed in breast self-examination, and had regular mammography according to the American Cancer Society guidelines. Whenever breast cancer was discovered in one of his patients, he made sure to inform her of the diagnosis personally and in as compassionate a manner as possible. Convinced that his surgical colleagues did not have the time for and interest in the patient that he did, he also made the skin incision for the surgery each patient would subsequently undergo.

When the general surgeon who performed most of the breast surgery in this community saw one of the internist's patients for the first time with the skin incision ready made and steri-stripped closed, he was mildly surprised and inclined to take offense. "Why does he bother to send the patient to me if he thinks he can do the surgery himself?" However, the incision was well made and entirely appropriate, so he kept his mouth closed, performed the surgery, and everyone was happy. Over the years, however, he saw several patients whose skin incisions he considered suboptimal. In these cases, he faced the dilemma of performing the surgery in a manner he considered less than ideal or of telling the patient that the internist's incision was inappropriate. On the occasions when he started to tell the patient something of this sort, he immediately realized that the patients had total confidence in the correctness of anything their doctor did and that challenging the internist's abilities and judgment would prove counterproductive. So, in almost every case, he continued to perform breast surgery through a skin incision made by the internist.

Then one day he saw a young woman sent by the internist for mastectomy, with the usual skin incision steri-stripped closed on her chest. However, in this patient, no fine-needle aspirate of the lesion had been performed. The mammogram had shown a suspicious lesion, but when the surgeon compared it with previous mammograms that had been unavailable when the patient was first seen by the internist, the lesion had been present and unchanged for several years. The surgeon asked the hospital's most experienced mammographer to review the case. The mammographer concluded that the lesion had been present for years and should simply be followed with regular annual mammograms.

Now the surgeon had a real dilemma. He had a woman in his office, skin already incised, who thought she had breast cancer and needed a mastectomy. Now he realized he should have spoken frankly to the internist years ago and told him that he had no business doing skin incisions for breast surgery. By his silence, he had collaborated in the sequence of events that had led to the mistake sitting his office today. What was he going to do?

To Earnest Souls

Some say an acorn is not an oak
And sapling but shadow of the elm

One so small it wraps upon itself
hard and unknowing
invulnerable to cold and drought alike
untouched by worlds beyond
an island sufficient unto itself
itself alone

Sapling branches out into the world
but is victim of the wind
each gust makes it kneel
in homage to greater power
as it weakly tries to gain the sinews
of elms

What gives you faith small tree?
frail child of such great company
to stand against the bitter threat
no strength to call your own
of torrents and ignominy
Is it the hope of majesty?

How easily your brother stands
how difficult for you
yet gracefully yielding to each assault
and righting yourself anew
Would that each man possess
your courage to progress

Then might the Lord be pleased
At a race of men as valiant as the trees

Martha Harwit, MD